An Atlas of
MULTIPLE PREGNANCY
Biology and Pathology

THE ENCYCLOPEDIA OF VISUAL MEDICINE SERIES

An Atlas of
MULTIPLE PREGNANCY
Biology and Pathology

Geoffrey A. Machin, MD, PhD

Regional Fetal Genetic Pathologist, The Permanente Medical Group,
Northern California Region, Oakland, and Visiting Professor of Pathology,
University of California at Davis, California

Louis G. Keith, MD

Professor of Obstetrics and Gynecology, Northwestern University Medical School and
President, The Center for the Study of Multiple Birth, Chicago, Illinois

With contributions from

Fiona Bamforth, MD

Department of Laboratory Medicine, University of Alberta Hospital, Edmonton, Alberta, Canada

David Teplica, MD, MFA

Department of Surgery, University of Chicago, Chicago, Illinois

Forewords by

John J. Sciarra, MD, PhD

Thomas J. Watkins Professor and Chairman, Department of Obstetrics and Gynecology,
Northwestern University Medical School, Chicago, Illinois

Emile Papiernik, MD

Professor of Obstetrics and Gynecology, Université René Descartes, Paris, France

The Parthenon Publishing Group
International Publishers in Medicine, Science & Technology

NEW YORK   LONDON

Library of Congress Cataloging-in-Publication Data
Machin, Geoffrey A.
    An atlas of multiple pregnancy : biology and pathology / Geoffrey
A. Machin, Louis G. Keith : with contributions from Fiona Bamforth
and David Teplica : forewords by John J. Sciarra, Emile Papiernik.
        p. cm. -- (The Encyclopedia of visual medicine series)
    Includes bibliographical references and index.
    ISBN 1-85070-918-1
    1. Multiple pregnancy--Atlases. I. Keith, Louis G. II. Title. III. Series.
    [DNLM: 1. Pregnancy, Multiple--atlases. WQ 17 M149a 1997]
RG567.M33 1997
618.2'5--dc21
DNLM/DLC
for Library of Congress   97-20395
                                                                          CIP

British Library Cataloguing-in-Publication Data
Machin, Geoffrey A.
    An atlas of multiple pregnancy : biology and pathology. -
    (The encyclopedia of visual medicine series)
    1. Multiple pregnancy - Atlases
I. Title II. Keith, Louis G. (Louis Gerald), 1935-
III. Bamforth, Fiona IV. Teplica, David
618.2'5
ISBN 1-85070-918-1

Published in the USA by
The Parthenon Publishing Group Inc.
One Blue Hill Plaza
PO Box 1564, Pearl River
New York 10965, USA

Published in the UK and Europe by
The Parthenon Publishing Group Limited
Casterton Hall, Carnforth
Lancs. LA6 2LA, UK

Copyright © 1999 Parthenon Publishing Group

First published 1999

Printed and bound in Spain by T.G. Hostench, S.A.

Contents

Foreword

Some years ago, I suggested that Professor Louis Keith was a wonderful *accoucheur* of textbooks. The passing years have definitely not caused me to change my mind. Now, as then, with this book, an authoritative collaboration has been formed. This time, however, it is Professor Geoffrey Machin, a pathologist of extraordinary experience and insight, who has taken the lead. The result of this partnership is more than admirable. Indeed, *An Atlas of Multiple Pregnancy* is eminently readable and has succeeded in presenting solid information elegantly.

For some time, clinicians have recognized a state of considerable confusion regarding the diagnosis of zygosity. The same may be said for twin–twin transfusion syndrome, a subject that has been misunderstood for more than a century. The syndrome is a rare occurrence and the pathophysiology underlying the condition is not easily described.

This has now all been changed with the routine use of ultrasonography to assess fetal wellbeing. However, what was still needed was a rational explanation for the combination of the clinical and pathophysiological states, and clear straightforward illustrations that were understandable to practicing clinicians.

Without doubt, this atlas provides exactly that – and much more – in a clear and concise text, and with a wealth of magnificent illustrations.

I am pleased that Machin and Keith have presented their work as a joint effort between the disciplines of pathology and obstetrics. These two branches have enjoyed a number of fruitful collaborations in the past, and this atlas is a noteworthy continuation of this long and great tradition.

Emile Papiernik
Paris

Foreword

As Professors Machin and Keith cogently note in their preface to this atlas of multiple pregnancy, the subject of twins is not new. However, their treatment of the topic is not only new, but unique. Both authors are internationally renowned in their respective fields – fetal pathology in the case of Geoffrey Machin, and multiple gestation in the case of Louis Keith. Working together for the first time as coauthors, they blend their talents in such a way that this book incorporates both of their points of view. This atlas contributes substantially to the body of scholarly works concerning multiple gestation by clarifying common misconceptions and providing clear guidelines to physicians regarding the early and accurate diagnosis of chorionicity and / or zygosity.

The text and figures are divided into three major sections. The first deals with 'classical' aspects of the topic with an emphasis on normality *vs* abnormality. The second section is a 'how to' guide written specifically to demystify the often repeated admonitions to clinicians on performing tests and examinations with which they may have little practical experience. To my knowledge, no other atlas is as equally directed to the learning needs of pathologists as well as clinicians. Finally, the third section on the lives of twins recreates the joys as well as some of the difficulties that accompany the accurate or inaccurate diagnosis of zygosity.

The atlas contains information that has been painstakingly gathered by Professor Machin during a career devoted to fetal pathology as well as concepts which, although previously described in the literature, have here been clarified anew by Professor Keith's sharp editorial pen. In view of the trend towards rising numbers of multiple births throughout the world, this volume will enhance the care provided to mothers of multiples. As with Louis Keith's earlier book (*Multiple Pregnancy: Epidemiology, Gestation and Perinatal Outcome*), this unique atlas should be of benefit to a wide audience of clinicians, medical students, parents and, of course, twins themselves.

John J. Sciarra
Chicago

Dedication

To my colleagues who shared their cases;
and to the twins and their families who have contributed
their knowledge and experience towards the creation of this book.

Geoffrey A. Machin

To my brother Donald, who for 41 years was my dizygotic ('fraternal') twin
and who, through the application of blood tests, then became my
monozygotic ('identical') twin brother. This transformation was wrought by
Professor Walter Nance and brought us closer together than we ever dreamed possible.
Our original blood grouping analysis has recently been reinforced by
state-of-the-art DNA testing.

Louis G. Keith

Preface

Twinning has long held a special place in the human imagination. Despite this, there are numerous misunderstandings about the condition of twinning. Most often, confusion is centered around the nature of the different types of twins and how they are formed. This atlas discusses some of the more recent advances in knowledge of the biology and pathology of twins and higher-order multiple pregnancies. With this book, we intend to clarify a number of areas of concern and interest to members of the healthcare professions as well as the general population.

As far as we are aware, much of the material in this book has never before been synthesized into a coherent whole. The study of twins overlaps such diverse fields as epidemiology, assisted reproduction, obstetrics, neonatology, medical genetics and psychology, to name but a few. Unlike other authors, we view twins as a coherent yet multifaceted area of study that is partially hidden, subtle and challenging at the very least. To this extent, *An Atlas of Multiple Pregnancy* is unique.

The number of twin and higher-order multiple pregnancies has increased dramatically throughout the world during the last ten years. In the United States, one in 45 pregnancies is now a twin or multiple pregnancy. This increase is primarily, but not exclusively, related to the increasing use of techniques to overcome infertility and to the older age of mothers at the time of their first pregnancies. Neither natural nor assisted multiple conceptions are without risk to either mothers or their fetuses.

The study of twins helps greatly in addressing questions regarding the relative effects on human development of genetic constitution and acquired experience. Nonetheless, recent research shows that numerous areas of investigation in twins require further study in the light of an improved understanding of how monozygotic (so-called identical) twin pairs may be dissimilar because of either genetic or environmental causes.

Once the antenatal diagnosis of twinning has been made, the known high risks of multiple pregnancies are all too often overshadowed by an inappropriate enthusiasm. The inherent risks are especially high when twins share a common monochorionic placenta. Despite recent technological advances in prenatal as well as neonatal care, outcomes are less than optimal. This is particularly true if, early in pregnancy, insufficient attention is paid to determining the precise placental type and exact relationship of the chorions. Failure to provide watchful and expectant prenatal care may lead to fetal and / or neonatal death and / or severe complications.

The illustrations in this atlas document salient points in twin biology, and the risks and complications of multiple pregnancies. There are also photographs which highlight fascinating aspects of the lives of twins in terms of their placental (chorion) type and known or presumed zygosity.

Unlike other collaborations, the responsibility for each section was not apportioned between the two authors for their eventual mutual comments and review. Instead, we sat down together, and began by reviewing more than 2000 illustrations and discussing how they might be used in this atlas. These discussions led to detailed outlines for the text sections. Several 'how to' sections have been included in Part II to correct the omissions of other previous books which have exhorted physicians to perform specific tasks, but have not provided detailed guidelines for their execution. Examples of such additions include how to examine twin placentas and make clinicopathological correlations, how to prepare optimal histological sections for chorionicity and zygosity determinations, how to test zygosity using DNA methodology and how to photograph twin faces for medical purposes.

Given this modus operandi, every page of text was edited by us together on screen so that the obstetrician could tell the pathologist what else he wanted to know, and the pathologist could revel in telling the obstetrician what he had missed. This was hard work, but it was wonderful fun.

This atlas also contains graphic documentation of the special aspects of twin biology and pathology that are more easily understood by illustration than by verbal description. In fact, the methods for investigating twin phenomena are disarmingly simple. The understanding of twins and their health care would be much improved if such methods were to be used more widely by both obstetricians and pathologists. Ultimately, it may well be that twins and their families will be the best advocates for some of the protocols put forward in this book.

The text and illustrations contained in this volume were compiled in Edinburgh when the senior author (GAM) was on sabbatical leave from the University of Alberta. This visiting professorship was facilitated by colleagues in the Medical Research Council Human Genetics Unit in Edinburgh, and by a Detweiler Travelling Fellowship awarded by the Royal College of Physicians and Surgeons of Canada. We have both received much support from our respective academic institutions and affiliations (The Permanente Medical Group, Northern California Region, and Northwestern University Medical School and the Center for Study of Multiple Birth, Chicago). In addition, various twins and their families have contributed their photographs and served as stimuli for the writing of specific portions of this book. Finally, we sincerely appreciate the efforts of Sharyn Wong, project editor, and Lynda Payne, medical artist, of Parthenon Publishing, in bringing this book to fruition.

We believe that this atlas will be useful to a wide variety of healthcare professionals. Epidemiologists and medical geneticists should find this book to be of particular value because of the sections dealing with twin biology. In addition, the parents or expectant parents of multiples may find useful information here to dispel the common misunderstandings that surround the special processes unique to multiple pregnancy, and to prepare them for the manifold joys and occasional sorrows that may accompany multiple births.

Readers will undoubtedly notice our deliberate selection of an italic typeface for emphasis. In addition, a few sentences are set in capital letters as a means of denoting their particular importance.

Geoffrey A. Machin
Louis G. Keith
Oakland and Chicago

Part 1 GENERAL ASPECTS

Glossary

$a \leftrightarrow a$	arterioarterial	**MZ**	monozygotic
AFP	alpha-fetoprotein	**PBT**	polar-body twinning
ART	assisted reproductive technology	**PI**	pulsatility index
$a \rightarrow v$	arteriovenous	**QA**	quadra-amniotic
DA	diamniotic	**RFLP**	restriction fragment length polymorphism
DC	dichorionic	**TA**	triamniotic
DZ	dizygotic	**TC**	trichorionic
FSH	follicle-stimulating hormone	**TRAP**	twin reversed arterial perfusion
HOMP	higher-order multiple pregnancy	**TTT**	twin–twin transfusion
IVF	*in vitro* fertilization	**TZ**	trizygotic
MA	monoamniotic	**VNTR**	variable number tandem repeat
MC	monochorionic	$v \leftrightarrow v$	venovenous
MSAFP	maternal serum alpha-fetoprotein		

Section 1 Biology of twins and other multiple pregnancies

Epidemiology

The frequency of natural twin pregnancy varies with maternal age, race, nutritional status, environment, season of conception and point in historical time. In recent years, various types of assisted reproductive technologies (ART) have greatly increased the total frequency of multiple pregnancies. Spontaneously conceived multiples occur most frequently in Nigeria, where the majority of such births are dizygotic (DZ), the result of more than one simultaneous ovulation. Each egg is fertilized by one sperm. The frequency of spontaneous multiple pregnancy is lowest in Japan, where almost two-thirds of multiple births are monozygotic (MZ) wherein a single fertilized egg gives rise to twins.

Despite these apparently dramatic differences, the prevalence of naturally conceived MZ twins is relatively constant worldwide, and differences in the overall rate of twinning are due to variable frequencies in the prevalence of DZ twins (Table 1.1). The prevalence of twins and higher-order

multiple pregnancies (HOMPs) has increased markedly in countries where various forms of ART are available. Ovulation-induction therapies and *in vitro* fertilization (IVF), the two main types of ART, both result in large numbers of HOMPs. In recent years, selective reduction has been offered to some mothers with triplets and higher-order gestations primarily because of the very high risks of preterm delivery and / or medical complications associated with these pregnancies.

Naturally conceived MZ twins occur with a frequency of approximately 3.5 / 1000 births. For reasons that are currently unknown, around 10–12% of pregnancies conceived after ART also result in MZ twins. In addition, some higher-order pregnancies, for example, quadra- and quinta- zygotic pregnancies, may contain MZ twins or triplets. The celebrated Dionne quintuplets were MZ.

Standard texts often propose that roughly 1 in 80 pregnancies results in twins, but this rate of incidence is based on outmoded assumptions. Recent calculations using data from the 1990 US census show that the frequency is, in fact, around 1 in 43 births. In the racially mixed USA population, roughly 30–40% of naturally conceived twins are MZ and 60–70% are DZ. These proportions are reversed in Japan. According to Hellin's law, postulated early in this century, spontaneous triplet pregnancies occur in 1 in 80^2 gestations or $1:6400$, and spontaneous quadruplets in 1 in 80^3 or $1:512\,000$ gestations. These figures are now only of historical interest, yet are often quoted by the popular press in the absence of population-based data.

Table 1.1 Relative worldwide frequencies of naturally conceived monozygotic (MZ) and dizygotic (DZ) twins

Country / race	DZ / 100 gestations	MZ (%)
Japan / Japanese	2.3	60
Hong Kong / Chinese	6.8	34
Great Britain / White	8.9	31
South Africa / Bantu	17.5	17
Nigeria / Yoruba	44.5	7

NB: These calculations assume a constant worldwide prevalence of MZ twins at 3.5 / 1000 gestations

The frequency of spontaneous twinning has also increased in recent years, especially in mothers who give birth after age 35 years. The importance of twin pregnancies to health care is twofold. First, their likelihood of preterm birth (<37 weeks of gestation) is nine to ten times greater than in singleton pregnancies. In addition, a disproportionate number (around ten times more than with singletons) are of extremely low birth weight (< 1500 g). As a result, preterm and / or low birth-weight twins (and higher-order multiples) spend significant amounts of time in neonatal intensive care units, often consuming scarce budgetary resources. *Second, the majority (around two-thirds) of MZ twins are connected to a single, monochorionic (MC) placenta, and are at risk of serious and potentially life-threatening complications. Major adverse consequences may derive from the blood vessels that connect an MC pair across their common placenta (see below).*

Table 1.2 Gestational age at delivery and perinatal mortality in twins analyzed by chorionicity and zygosity

Placentation, zygosity	Gestational age (weeks) at delivery (%)			
	20–27	28–35	>35	Total
Fused, DZ (DC)	4	41	55	100
Separate, DZ (DC)	5	32	63	100
All DZ	5	36	59	100
Fused, DC, MZ	0	39	61	100
Separate, DC, MZ	0	50	50	100
All DC, MZ	0	43	57	100
All DC (DZ, MZ)	4	38	58	100
MZ, MC	15	45	41	100
All MZ (DC, MC)	11	44	45	100
All twins	8	40	52	100

Placentation, zygosity	Perinatal mortality (%)
MZ, MC	16
MZ, DC	1
DZ (DC)	11

DZ, dizygotic; DC, dichorionic; MZ, monozygotic; MC, monochorionic

Data derived from Machin *et al.* Some perinatal characteristics of monozygotic twins who are dichorionic. *Am J Med Genet* 1995;55:71–6

The statistics for morbidity and mortality are particularly high for the MC / MZ subgroup of twins compared with dichorionic (DC) twins, regardless of MZ or DZ status (Table 1.2, lower panel).

Zygosity and related issues

MZ compared with DZ twin types

MZ twins occur when one fertilized egg gives rise to two embryos. It is not known how or why this happens, although there are data regarding the general timing of the event(s) (see below). Fertilization of an aging ovum may be an important predisposing factor. MZ twins are rarely familial (see Part III), and the cause of familial MZ twinning is yet to be investigated.

Contrary to conventional expectations, MZ twins are rarely absolutely identical. Most often, they are extremely similar. Occasionally, they may look dissimilar either because of different genetic constitutions or as a result of different environmental influences, some of which may be prenatal (see below).

DZ twins arise when the mother ovulates two eggs in the same cycle, often one from each ovary, and both are fertilized. It is probable that DZ twinning is caused by higher-than-normal levels of follicle-stimulating hormone (FSH) or by an exaggerated response to FSH, with the result that more than one egg is ovulated from among the several that ripen in a given cycle. This tendency is heritable and accounts for the familial occurrence of DZ twins. There may be a gene for DZ twinning, and large families with high frequencies of DZ twins are currently under investigation to determine the presence of such a gene. Ethnic / racial variations in the frequency of DZ twinning can be explained in the same way. By chance, it would be expected that half of all DZ twins would be like-sexed and half would be unlike-sexed.

DZ twins may have one father (homopaternity) or different fathers (heteropaternity). Heteropaternity (involving superfecundation) is probably rare. Homopaternal DZ twins have the usual degree of familial likeness commonly seen in siblings with the same parents. In contrast, heteropaternal DZ twins exhibit varying degrees of dissimilarity to the extent of even having different racial origins. On occasions, homopaternal DZ twins are remarkably similar, thereby raising the possibility that they are in fact MZ. This question can only be answered by definitive zygosity testing (see Part II, Section 2). It is unlikely that human twins are conceived in different cycles but, should such superfetation occur, it should not be confused with true twinning.

Considerations of nature and nurture in relation to twin zygosity

In the classical twin model, it is assumed that MZ twin pairs emerge 'innocent' or 'untouched', having experienced similar prenatal environments and inherited the same genetic constitutions. In this paradigm, major likenesses in later life must be genetically determined and major differences must be due to different postnatal experiences. In contrast, similarities in DZ twins are presumed to be the result of similar environments during childhood whereas differences are then reflections of varying genetic constitutions. This neat, tidy and widely accepted *tabula rasa* or 'clean-slate' construct is now known to be an oversimplification. Clearly, on occasions, MZ twins may have different genetic constitutions, although the frequency of such occurrences is not yet known.

It has recently been suggested that subtle, yet discrete, genetic differences among groups of cells arising within the early embryo may, in fact, initiate or stimulate the twinning process by causing separation of the genetically distinct cell clusters (Figure 1.1, pages 96–7). Whether or not this is the cause of MZ twinning, it is clear that MZ twins often experience different antenatal environments, particularly through unequal sharing of nutrients or because of vascular interactions in MC placentas.

DZ twins may also experience different antenatal environments, including unfavorable or even heterotopic sites of placental implantation for one twin. Different intrapartum environmental experiences may occur in MZ as well as DZ twins (see Figure 1.1), for example, acute intrapartum twin-to-twin transfusion in MC, MZ twins, and discordant intrapartum human immunodeficiency virus (HIV) infection of MZ and DZ twins during passage through the birth canal.

A final consideration of the nature/nurture construct relates to the fact that some MZ twins appear, over time, to come to resemble each other more closely rather than becoming more discordant. It is possible that genetically determined behaviors may cause the twins to perceive, select and experience similar environments, thereby reinforcing their similarities. This may be particularly true of MZ twins who are raised apart. (Indeed, it has been noted that many pairs of MZ twins raised apart appear to resemble each other even more closely that do those pairs who are raised together.) In contrast, specific antenatal environmental influences may cause discordance. Thus, just as there can be "many a slip 'twixt cup and lip", so are there many factors that can cause MZ twin pairs to be phenotypically distinct at birth (see Figure 1.1).

Despite these caveats, there is much evidence to suggest that MZ twin pairs are usually genetically close to identical and that this fact has a major influence on their postnatal physical as well as psychological development. Apart from the results of classical long-term follow-up studies, there is additional tangential evidence in support of the importance of genetic influences. This derives from newer studies of MZ twin pairs who were adopted at birth, separated and raised in different environments. As adults, these twin pairs generally show striking physical, mental and psychological similarities.

Polar-body twinning (PBT)

During normal ovulation, most of the cytoplasm is retained by the cell that contains the nucleus and normally forms the single egg. If, by chance, sufficient cytoplasm segregates with the nuclei of either the first or second polar body, this structure may then be capable of becoming fertilized. It has also been suggested that the ovum may undergo further cell division in the haploid state prior to or during fertilization, giving rise to monovular DZ twins. Such twins would differ in their paternally derived genes, but have the same or similar maternally derived genes. Thus, their genetic constitutions would be in between those of MZ and DZ twins. However, this is not the case in PBT (Figure 1.2, page 98) because polar bodies and their corresponding ova are not genetically identical.

Many parents have difficulty in understanding how their MZ twins can be so similar in appearance, yet so easily distinguishable physically and psychologically by those who know the twins well. Indeed, their 'identical' twins are merely MZ. In such circumstances, parents may erroneously conclude that their offspring are PBT.

It is entirely reasonable to question whether close similarities are caused by identical maternal genetic contributions via PBT. However, if twins were to be derived from an ovum and its first polar body, they would, in fact, be less alike than DZ twins. Thus, the rare phenomenon of PBT is probably not the true explanation for the vast majority of MZ twins who are very similar, but not identical in every aspect from alpha to omega.

The rank order of genetic similarity in the types of twin pairs is: first PBT < DZ < second PBT < uniovular dispermatic < MZ.

More research is needed to validate the existence of the two possible types of PBT. In the only well-studied pair of twins with evidence of PBT, one twin was diploid and the other was triploid; this pair had apparently resulted from a failure to produce a second polar body at the second meiotic division. Therefore, they were not a product of PBT *per se*. Indeed, as the only documented example of PBT has been diploid and triploid, they cannot be considered an example of close twin similarity!

Timing of MZ twinning events

The timing of twinning can be inferred from the structure of the placenta, membranes and yolk sac(s). The earlier the twinning event, the greater is the degree to which each embryo is provided with adequate extraembryonic structures. Embryos that are formed early are therefore more autonomous and physiologically independent than those resulting from later twinning events.

At around 2 days postconception (pc), progenitor cells of the zygote become specialized and separate into two cell populations: one group (the outer cell mass) forms the placenta; the other (the inner cell mass) gives rise to the body of the embryo. Different types of placentation result, depending on the timing of the MZ twinning event in relation to the separation of these two cell groups (Figure 1.3, page 99). *If twinning takes place prior to day 2 pc, two complete placentas and two sets of membranes are formed, one for each embryo. This subset of MZ twins are dichorionic (DC), as are all DZ twins (Figure 1.4, page 99). Approximately one-third of MZ twins are DC.* Each placental disk may remain separate or the two may grow sufficiently close to one another that they fuse.

At around 2 days pc, the progenitor cells of the placenta (trophoblast) become separated from the inner cell mass of the embryo. *If the MZ twinning event occurs between 2 and 8 days pc, only one placenta is programmed to develop. This single placenta is MC, diamniotic (DA), and caters to the nutritional needs of both embryos. Approximately two-thirds of MZ twins have MC placentas. These placentas are more similar to placentas supporting singleton fetuses than to fused DC placentas except in one important respect: the circulations of the MZ twin pair frequently meet and mingle on the surface and in the substance of the placenta (see Figure 1.4).* Such a fateful happenstance occurs very rarely, if ever, in fused DC placentas, and a shared circulation clearly represents a major cause of complications in MC, MZ twins (see below).

At around 8 days pc (see Figure 1.3), the amniotic ectoderm and cavity separate from the rest of the embryo. *If the twinning process occurs after 8 days pc, the MZ twin pair share a common amniotic sac as well as an MC placenta; they are monoamniotic (MA). Approximately 5% of MZ twins are MC, MA.* The yolk sac forms at about this time. MC, DA twins have two yolk sacs whereas MC, MA twins have only one. The frequency of these events in relation to timing and placentation, based on reports of large series of twins from several tertiary medical centers, is shown in Table 1.3.

Finally, at around 12–13 days pc, the main cranio-caudal axis of the embryo is laid down. *It is believed that conjoined twinning occurs at or around this time.* Paradoxically, the twins who are most closely associated with each other are the result of partial splitting at the last possible moment, after which

Table 1.3 Placentation in twins

Author	DC, DA (%)	MC, DA (%)	MC, MA (%)
Benirschke, 1961	69	30	1.0
Potter, 1993	76	21	3.0
Cameron, 1968	80	20	0.0
Fujikura, 1971	73	24	2.4
Barss, 1988	74	14	2.0

time the zygote would have retained its singleton status.

Because all MC twins are MZ by definition and all unlike-sexed twins are DZ by definition, the zygosity of 55% of all twins can be determined at birth without the use of special techniques. In contrast, the zygosity of twin pairs who are like-sexed and DC requires specific zygosity testing for determination (Figure 1.5, page 100; see also Part II, Section 2).

As noted above, spontaneously conceived HOMPs consist of combinations of MZ and DZ twinning events, *but with a high proportion of MZ twinning.* Numerous varieties of placental arrangements are found. The same is true with purely MZ HOMPs, depending on the timing of the successive twinning events. Possible combinations for MZ triplet placentation are shown diagrammatically in Figure 1.6, page 100.

Whereas an understanding of placental anatomy offers information on the timing of MZ twinning events, it does not clarify the nature of these events. *All MZ twins with MC placentas, whether DA, MA or conjoined, are associated with a high risk of gestational complications because of the specific anatomical arrangements of the placental blood vessels.* Although the chorionicity of twins can be diagnosed with considerable accuracy by early obstetric ultrasound, in clinical practice, this early distinction between DC and MC twins is not made universally.

Mechanisms of MZ twinning

The mechanisms underlying MZ twinning still await clarification. Regardless of whether or not MZ twinning is considered an example of abnormal embryogenesis (probably with high rates of antenatal embryo / fetal loss), the proposed mechanisms leading to MZ twinning fall into two main classes.

Extrinsic causes

Extrinsic causes resemble the situation in IVF where manipulation of the egg causes premature rupture of the zona pellucida, resulting in spillage of part of the early embryo. This circumstance may cause physical separation of two early cell masses, leading to the formation of MZ twins. If this process were to occur spontaneously, it could also cause some of the more severe forms of congenital anomalies seen in MZ twins, such as amniotic band syndrome or parasitic conjoined twins.

Intrinsic postzygotic differences

On the other hand, intrinsic postzygotic differences among the cells of the inner cell mass may lead to aggregation of similar cells into two or more groups. These groups may be subsequently driven apart by mutual recognition and repulsion, resulting in the formation of genetically distinct MZ twins. Such twin pairs would be remarkable because of their marked phenotypic dissimilarities.

Postzygotic chromosomal non-disjunction

There are several ways in which MZ twins may be discordant because of genetic constitution or maldevelopment. Postzygotic chromosomal non-disjunction produces mosaicism in those singletons who have two cell lines of different chromosomal constitutions derived from one zygote. These events may also occur in embryos destined to become MZ twins. It is not known whether such events in fact cause twinning, but it is certainly plausible, as numerous MZ twin pairs of different chromosomal constitution have been reported (Table 1.4). The degree of phenotypic dissimilarity may extend as far as different external genitalia. For example, in a twin pair derived from a 46,XY zygote, one was a normal 46,XY male and the other was a 45,X Ullrich–Turner phenotypic female.

Hypothetically, through two different postzygotic sex-chromosome non-disjunctions, it is possible for 47,XXY zygotes to give rise to MZ twins with different sex-chromosome constitutions, including a chromosomally normal female (46,XX) and a chromosomally normal male (46,XY; Figure 1.7, page 101).

In cases in which a trisomic zygote returns to diploid euploidy through postzygotic loss of one of the trisomic chromosomes, considerations of parental origin of the extra chromosome become relevant (see Figure 1.7). In the case of second meiotic non-disjunction, one parent contributes two copies of the same set of alleles (uniparental isodisomy; see Figure 1.7). If one of these alleles is a mutant form of a recessive gene, two types of postzygotic events could result in an MZ twin pair discordant for a recessive disease.

X-chromosome inactivation

X-chromosome inactivation is a further important postzygotic mechanism that may on occasions be involved in the twinning process (Figure 1.8, pages 102–3). There is an excess of females among MZ

Table 1.4 Chromosomal discordance in monozygotic twin pairs

Twin A	Twin B
45,X	46,XY
45,X	46,XX
45,X	46,X idic (Y)
21 trisomy	normal
18 trisomy	normal
13 trisomy	normal
46,XY / 46,X,-Y,+der (Y)	46,XY
46,XX,-13,r13	46,XX
46,XY,del (7)	46,XY
46,XY,del (10)	46,XY

twins, and the excess increases the later the twinning event, such that 75% of conjoined twins are female. Therefore, it is possible that X-chromosome inactivation may in some way be causally linked to the MZ twinning process in females.

Several pairs of MZ female twins have been noted to be discordant for genetic diseases of X-linked type (for example, Duchenne muscular dystrophy; see Table 1.5). The pattern of X-chromosome inactivation is skewed in the affected twin, with an excess of inactivated X chromosomes bearing the normal allele. In contrast, the phenotypically normal co-twin may show random X-chromosome inactivation or an inactivation pattern which is skewed in the opposite direction to that of the co-twin. It is not yet clear whether this event may in fact cause twinning or merely represents a result of the MZ twinning process.

Analysis of patterns of X-chromosome inactivation in female twins without X-linked disease shows that markedly skewed X-chromosome inactivation is rarely seen. Skewed inactivation appears to be limited to those special cases where the X chromosome bears a mutant gene on one allele. In female MZ pairs with skewed / normal patterns of X-chromosome inactivation, analysis of the size of clones of cells with opposite X-chromosome inactivation suggests that the affected twin may have arisen from a smaller number of progenitor cells than the normal twin. This is evidence that the allocation of blastomeres to a pair of twins is not necessarily equal. This, in turn, has important implications for the etiology of several diseases that are found only in MZ twin pairs.

Differential gene imprinting

Differential gene imprinting may account for several pairs of MZ twins who have been found to be discordant for the phenotypic expression of Beckwith–Wiedemann syndrome (Figure 1.9, page 104).

Discordance for autosomal single-gene disease

Discordance for autosomal single-gene disease has only been convincingly reported in one MZ twin pair. Many cases of autosomal-dominant disease arise by *de novo* mutation, usually in a parental germ line. However, it is to be expected that discordance for autosomal-dominant disease may be reported in MZ twin pairs where the mutation has occurred after fertilization.

Special consideration is given to those genes which contain trinucleotide repeats (as seen in, for example, X-linked mental retardation or Huntington's disease). Preliminary work shows that, within MZ twin pairs, there are demonstrable small differences in the expansion repeat numbers; these differences represent postzygotic (not meiotic) events which could therefore cause discrepancy in the severity of expression of this type of disease in MZ twin pairs.

Discordance for major malformations

Discordance for major malformations is also seen in MZ twin pairs (Figure 1.10, page 105). Such malformations include neural tube defect, cleft lip and palate, omphalocele, congenital heart disease, holoprosencephaly and symmelia. The cause of such discordance is not known at present. *From the practical point of view, it is important to recognize that twin pairs discordant for major malformations are not necessarily DZ, but may well be MZ and, more*

Table 1.5 Results of skewed X-inactivation in female MZ twin pairs

X-linked mental retardation

Duchenne muscular dystrophy

Red-green color blindness

Hunter syndrome

Fabry disease

important, MC. Antenatal diagnosis of discordant malformation may lead to consideration of selective termination, but this procedure requires special precautions in cases of MZ, MC pairs.

These unusual and often misunderstood examples of discordant twin pairs are important in the appreciation of the complex nature of the MZ twinning process. They particularly highlight the fact that the allocation of blastomeres to the inner cell masses of MZ twins may be clearly unequal. In reality, there is no reason to assume that blastomere allocation is invariably equal. Indeed, unequal allocation may underlie a number of disease processes in MZ twins, including 'vanishing' twins, acardius and twin-to-twin transfusion syndrome. What is clear is that all MZ twin pairs must complete an extra mitotic cell cycle to achieve the same body size as DZ twins and singletons. As many developmental processes are closely related to timing (and possibly to the number of cell divisions achieved) after conception, MZ twins are probably at an increased risk for maldevelopment on this basis alone.

Placentas of twins

The number of placentas is commonly believed by healthcare workers, parents and twins themselves to equate directly with zygosity. This premise is only partially correct; newborn like-sexed twins are often erroneously diagnosed as DZ simply because they each have one placenta (DC), whether separate or fused. The number of sacs, unless specified by chorionicity, is imprecise **per se** *and, in fact, may lead to important misinformation (see Part III, Misassignment of zygosity at birth).*

DZ twins always develop one placenta each; therefore, they are always DC. These placentas may fuse as they grow if they are implanted close together (Figure 1.11 a, page 106); if they implant sufficiently far apart within the uterus, they will remain separate (Figure 1.11 b, page 106). In contrast, MZ twins

may have either one (MC) or two placentas (DC; Figures 1.11 c & d, page 107), depending on the timing of the twinning event (see above and Figure 1.3).

The relationships between zygosity and placental anatomy shown in Figure 1.11 e (page 108) refer to a typical white European–North American population of spontaneously conceived twins, among whom approximately 70% are DZ and 30% are MZ. DC placentas of MZ twins are more frequently fused than those of DZ twins, presumably because they issue from the same Fallopian tube. *It is commonly and mistakenly assumed that all twins with DC placentation are DZ. However, DC placentas provide no information whatsoever on zygosity in like-sexed twin pairs, in contrast to MC placentas, which always denote MZ twinning.*

Fused DC placentas possess membranous septa consisting of four layers: two layers of chorion and two layers of amnion (DC, DA). This anatomical arrangement acts as a barrier to prevent any contact between the circulations of the twins, even in cases of fused DC, MZ placentas (see Figure 1.4). Each twin is an independent physiological unit and does not significantly impinge on the cardiovascular system of the other.

MC placentas, in contrast, most commonly have a single disk, although two separate disks are occasionally present (see Part I, Section 3, *Anatomy of monochorionic twin placentas*). MC placentas with a single disk are no different in structure from the solitary placentas of singletons – they do not represent fusion of separate structures.

Connections between the two fetal circulations are not only possible but frequent occurrences in MZ, MC gestations and, when present, can cause significant problems. *In the absence of a chorionic component in the septum between the two sacs, fetal blood vessels from both twins intermix on the surface of the single placenta and within its substance (see Figure 1.11 c). These anastomoses are largely responsible for many of the high risks associated with MC twin pregnancies.*

Ultrasound examination of septal membrane thickness is best carried out in the first trimester. The number of layers and, hence, the thickness of the membranous septum is a key issue in the early prenatal assessment of twin pregnancy. A thin septum (≤2 mm) may denote MC, DA twins with an increased risk of complications (see Part I, Section 2) whereas a thick septum (approximately 4 mm) usually denotes a DC, DA placenta with no associated risk of vascular communication. However, the presence of such a septum *per se* provides no information regarding zygosity. On rare occasions, a septum between the two fetuses is entirely absent; such placentation is monochorionic and monoamniotic (MC, MA; see Figure 1.11 d).

The various types of MZ placentation are shown in Figure 1.11 f (page 108). The two main types of vascular anastomoses with MC placentas (see above) are shown in Figure 1.12 (pages 109–10). *Both arterioarterial (a↔a) and venovenous (v↔v) connections occur on the chorionic surface of the placenta. In contrast, arteriovenous (a→v) connections occur only within the villous parenchyma of the placenta where the arterial supply to a specific villous region (cotyledon) derives from one twin, and the venous return is to the other. Such connections are not malformations, but merely abnormal arrangements resulting from the presence of two fetal circulations within a truly single placenta.* This fact has been known since the late nineteenth century, but is still not fully appreciated nor applied in clinical practice.

The a→v connections may be single or multiple, and may run in one or both directions. In general, the vascular anatomy of MC placentas is not complex. The overall frequency and combinations of vascular anastomoses are available in the literature.

The clinical importance of vascular anastomoses in MC placentas cannot be overemphasized (see Part I, Section 2, *Complications of monochorionic twin pregnancy*). These connections may cause a net transfusion of blood from one twin to the other, commonly referred to as twin–twin transfusion (TTT), which often leads to major complications. *TTT usually only occurs in the presence of deep (parenchymal) a→v anastomoses with no superficial a↔a or v↔v anastomoses to exert a protective and compensatory effect.*

Reproductive technology and multiple births

The prevalence of twins and higher-order multiple births has increased markedly since the introduction of medical therapies to overcome infertility. Because the rate of successful implantation of embryos is relatively low after IVF, many clinicians transfer multiple embryos in the hope that at least one will implant and result in a clinical pregnancy. However, this practice has resulted not only in increasing the singleton pregnancy rate, but has also contributed to the 'explosion' in the number of twin and higher-order pregnancies. A similar observation may be made as regards the use of ovulation-inducing agents.

Because of the extent of the risk associated with higher-order gestations, some countries, such as the United Kingdom, place strict limits on the number of embryos that can be replaced at any one time. Other countries, such as the USA, have no such restrictions, and pregnancy reduction is often offered to mothers of triplet or higher-order ART pregnancies.

When selective termination is offered, the practice has been aptly characterized as a treatment to counteract the effects of a treatment given to a patient to overcome infertility, a condition rather than a disease. The debate over the appropriateness of fetal reduction as a therapy is particularly poignant because the gestational age at delivery and survival rates of multiple pregnancy are inversely proportional to the degree of polyembryony.

Some reasons why monozygotic twins are not identical

In our experience, this question causes more confusion than any other in the understanding of twin biology. In particular, it is often difficult for twins and their parents to understand the difference between the term 'monozygotic', which is precise and correct, and the more commonly used term 'identical' which, not unreasonably, is presumed to mean 'absolutely identical'.

As already discussed in the section on the mechanisms of MZ twinning, there are more genetic and environmental reasons for MZ twins to be dissimilar than there are genetic reasons for them to be considered 'identical'. Therefore, it is strongly recommended that the latter term be avoided in the context of twins, especially when attempting to use accurate scientific terminology and / or to explain zygosity.

Phenotypic discordance in MZ twin pairs may be the result of one or both of two distinct processes, namely, the rare but precise genetic difference, or the much more common abnormal prenatal environment of the MC placenta. *In particular, unequal sharing of the placental parenchyma can lead to discordant birth weights and other dissimilarities even in the absence of TTT.* As another example, it is difficult to imagine a more phenotypically discordant twin pair than the acardiac twin and its pump co-twin (see Part I, Section 3, *Mechanisms of acardius*). Nevertheless, such twins are indeed MZ because they are MC.

Abnormal vascular events during gestation in MC twins may be associated with varying degrees of residual organ damage in one or both twins. A multitude of lesions, including cerebral, hepatic, pulmonary and renal infarction, intestinal atresias and aplasia cutis, are the result of hypoxic / hypotensive / ischemic episodes secondary to blood pressure fluctuations in the fetuses transmitted through interfetal placental vascular anastomoses. When only one twin is adversely affected, discordance results. If TTT is present, the smaller 'donor' twin is more likely to suffer from these events than the larger recipient co-twin.

Despite the lack of precise knowledge concerning the earliest events in MZ twinning, evidence from X-chromosome-inactivation studies suggests that unequal numbers of embryonic cells may be distributed to the two embryos and their corresponding parts of the placenta(s). These early abnormal events may also explain discordance for body growth and malformation in MZ twin pairs. For these reasons, the relationships between genotype, prenatal environment and placental anatomy are not straightforward in terms of determination of the eventual phenotype of MZ twin pairs. Few assumptions can be made, and careful thought has to be given to difficult cases before definite conclusions can be drawn. Some of the results of false assumptions concerning zygosity are further explored in Part III.

Twins in research

Prior oversimplification of the complexities of twin zygosity, chorionicity, genotype and phenotype has led to erroneous results in some twin studies. Several environmental and postzygotic antenatal genetic events, acting either alone or in concert, may result in MZ twin pairs who display a wide spectrum of phenotypic discordance at birth. To the casual observer, they thus appear more likely than not to be DZ.

Twin studies should not be considered complete without formal definitive zygosity determination. New cohorts of twins followed from birth should be enrolled with complete information on the zygosity, placentation and the differential phenotypic features, such as growth discordance, that are manifest at birth.

With such refinements of perinatal 'non-identity' in place, the power of twin studies will be greatly enhanced and will allow more discriminatory analysis of information than is currently available.

Section 2 Antepartum diagnosis and management of twin pregnancies

Introduction

In the era before ultrasound, the detection, prevention and / or active management of antenatal and intrapartum complications of multiple pregnancy were, at best, inadequate and, at worst, totally lacking. High rates of morbidity and mortality were common among twins. Although radiography was available, its value was limited. This situation was changed dramatically when ultrasound became widely available as a practical diagnostic tool.

At present, a significant percentage of pregnant women undergo at least one early ultrasound study for confirmation of gestational age. One of the principal benefits of such an assessment is the early diagnosis of twins and higher-order multiple pregnancies (HOMPs). Considerable diagnostic benefit is also obtained from the test screening for maternal serum alpha-fetoprotein (MSAFP). Originally introduced to detect lower-than-normal values as a possible indication of trisomic fetuses, it was soon noted that twin pregnancies are associated with abnormally high levels of MSAFP. However, as MSAFP levels are not absolutely diagnostic of twinning, further confirmation is required; for this, ultrasound is the test of choice.

As with singleton pregnancy, the ultimate clinical and economic benefits of ultrasound screening remain under intense scrutiny. Regardless of the final direction of this discussion, *the authors remain firmly convinced that ultrasound is invaluable in the early detection of twin and HOMP pregnancies, and their continued assessment.*

Early and accurate diagnosis of twin pregnancies and HOMPs has three specific benefits. First, the pregnancy can be immediately characterized as being at high risk for reasons already discussed (see Part I, Section 1). Parents can be advised of the need to take extra precautions as well as to seek early medical attention for unusual signs and symptoms. Although the frequency of preterm labor and delivery may or may not be reduced by recognition of the high-risk pregnancy status *per se*, there is little doubt that stillbirth and neonatal mortality rates decline when multiple pregnancy status is known.

Second, the natural history of HOMPs can be assessed more accurately. Such gestations are without doubt associated with even higher risks of preterm delivery than are twins. This risk can be reduced by intensive prenatal care (including selective fetal reduction) and also by efforts directed towards modifying the maternal lifestyle.

The third and least often accomplished benefit of ultrasound has the greatest potential value, namely, the early and unequivocal recognition of the nature of the septal membranes between the gestation sacs. *A clear distinction can usually be made between monochorionic (MC) and dichorionic (DC) pregnancies by early and accurate assessment of the thickness of the septal membranes and their structure as they arise from the placental surface (see below).*

With the knowledge that a twin pregnancy may be MC, obstetricians can inform their patients of the special types and degrees of risk in such pregnancies without causing unnecessary alarm. More important, medical caregivers can take appropriate steps to reduce the high frequency of poor outcomes (see Part III). It is paradoxical that this essential point is the one which is least understood and / or considered. Given that the diagnostic precision for delineating chorionicity decreases with gestational age, it is disappointing to note how infrequently this physical characteristic is fully described when ultrasound examinations are performed early in pregnancy.

Ultrasound also provides important information on the natural history of twin pregnacy, most notably by establishing the presence and frequency of the 'vanishing twin' and documenting the adverse consequences to the survivor if one twin dies *in utero*. In addition, ultrasound is effective in monitoring twin pregnancies for fetal wellbeing and detecting the serious consequences of MC placentation: TTT, twin reversed arterial perfusion (TRAP), growth discordance and fetal death. Finally, ultrasound is mandatory when complications are investigated and treated with interventive technologies such as amniocentesis, fetal surgery and selective fetal termination.

The following section refers to ultrasonograms from a number of published and unpublished sources, and illustrates important steps in the diagnosis and management of twin pregnancies as well as the prevention and treatment of various complications. However, it is not the intention of the authors to provide a comprehensive guide to ultrasonography. The reader is advised to refer to standard sources for further details.

External sexual differentiation

Fetal genitalia cannot be diagnosed with certainty until the mid-trimester (17–20 weeks). Unlike-sexed twins are virtually always DZ and therefore expected to be DC. There are rare exceptions to this 'rule', as in the case of postzygotic chromosome loss leading to MZ twin pairs with 46,XY and 45,X chromosome status, respectively (see Part I, Section 1 and Table 1.4). The 45,X fetus had female external genitalia and features of Ullrich–Turner syndrome. In contrast, like-sexed twins may be DZ (always DC) or MZ (MC or DC).

Number of placental disks

The number of placental disks is not specific for or diagnostic of either chorionicity or zygosity. *A small number of MC placentas have two disks or disks joined by small bridges of parenchymal tissue which may be overlooked on ultrasound* (see Part I, Section 3 and Figures 3.2 & 3.3). Large succenturiate lobes of MC placentas may also be mistaken for separate (DC) placental disks. The converse is equally true. *When an apparently single disk is present, it may be a truly single MC placenta or a fused DC placenta.*

Number of sacs

This information on its own has little value partly because 'sacs' refer to different structures at different gestational ages. In the first trimester, the presence of one or two gestational sacs may be obvious, as one or two complete chorionic structures may be seen, even if details within these sacs are not yet clear. Later in gestation, it may be apparent that each embryo lies within its own amniotic cavity, which is also commonly referred to as a 'sac'. It is far better, for clarity's sake, to refer to numbers of amnions and chorions, respectively.

Each fetus has its own (amniotic) cavity in the vast majority of twins and HOMPs. The finding of two such structures in twin pregnancies is highly likely, because MC, MA twins represent only around 1% of twins. There is little merit in merely stating that the twins are diamniotic, as the key issue is the number of chorions. Therefore, THE REAL QUESTION IS: *WHAT IS THE NATURE AND/OR STRUCTURE OF THE SEPTUM BETWEEN THE EMBRYOS?* (see *Number of embryos* below).

Structure of septal membranes and significance of the delta sign

The most important information required for the optimal management of multiple pregnancies depends on the early and accurate understanding of the structure of the septal membranes. This assessment is best carried out in the first trimester or early in the second trimester and preferably with the use of an endovaginal probe.

DC pregancies consist of two complete chorionic structures containing twins A and B, respectively. Each twin is surrounded by its own layers of chorion and amnion regardless of whether the placental disks are separate or fused. The septal membranes thus comprise four layers at the point where they meet or abut (Figure 2.1 a, page 111). In clinical practice, it is generally not possible to detect the four discrete layers individually. However, in the aggregate, the septa are substantial structures with a total thickness usually exceeding 4 mm (see Figure 2.1 a).

Equally important, the septal components of the chorion are attached to and contiguous with the placental chorionic plate at the junction of the septum and the placental surface. At this location, the two layers of chorion may diverge at the inferior margin to form a tent-like shape, variably characterized as the delta, lambda or twin-peak sign (Figure 2.1 b & c, pages 111–2). Although this sign occasionally persists as the gestation progresses, it is not always visible because the septum becomes thinner when the pressure of amniotic fluid flattens the area (Figure 2.1 d & e, pages 112–3).

In contrast to DC twin pregnancies, MC gestations are, by definition, surrounded by a single chorion, as in singleton pregnancies. Because the chorion (placenta) is truly single (not fused), the septum between MC, DA twins contains only amniotic components (Figure 2.2 a, page 113). Compared with the four-layered DC, DA septum, the two-layered MC, DA septum is insubstantial, and may be difficult to detect by ultrasound (Figure 2.2 b–d, pages 114–5) because it measures ≤2 mm in thickness. If the whole gestation is scanned, the septum is often seen inconsistently. A false-positive delta sign may sometimes be present (see Figure 2.2 c, page 114). Early in the first trimester, before the amnion can be visualized, the diagnosis of chorionicity can be made with confidence. However, given the difference in clinical outcomes between DC

and MC twins, it should not be considered a serious error to 'overdiagnose' as MC a pregnancy which later proves to be DC.

Around 5% of MC gestations are MC, MA (see Figure 1.11 e) and cannot be reliably diagnosed merely on the basis of failure to detect a septal membrane. The septum of an MC, DA pregnancy may be so thin that it falls below the limits of resolution, especially with the use of older equipment. In such instances, it is likely that a false-positive diagnosis of MC, MA placentation will be made. MC, DA twins have two yolk sacs whereas MC, MA twins have a single yolk sac (Figure 2.3 a, page 115). Circumstantial evidence obtained by repeat ultrasound examination may confirm true MC, MA status in some cases. If present, intertwined cords forming braids or the presence of conjoined twins are diagnostic of the MC, MA state.

Some investigators advocate the intra-amniotic injection of indigo–carmine dye or sterile air bubbles for computed tomography (CT) scanning to confirm the diagnosis of an MC, MA pregnancy (Figure 2.3 b, page 116). Methylene blue dye should never be used for this purpose because it can result in duodenal atresia and other problems. If the injected material spreads evenly throughout the gestational cavity and / or is taken up by both fetuses, then MA placentation is confirmed. If, on the other hand, the contrast material is limited to one-half of the gestational sac, then the presence of a septum is indicated (see Figure 2.3 b). On occasions, MC, DA pregnancies are converted into pseudomonoamniotic gestations either spontaneously, or by deliberate or inadvertent septal puncture during amniocentesis or other interventional procedures. This event may confuse the ultrasonographer and may have serious medical consequences.

It is recognized that septal membrane thickness and the delta sign are reliable methods for the diagnosis of chorion status. The examination is required not

Table 2.1 Consequences of antenatal misdiagnosis of chorionicity

Ultrasound diagnosis	Actual diagnosis	Consequence
MC	DC	not serious; can be downgraded later
DC	MC	may be serious; failure to anticipate early stages of TTT and other MC complications
MC, MA	MC, DA	not serious; can be downgraded later
MC, DA	MC, MA	may be serious; failure to anticipate conjoined twins, cord complications

MC, monochorionic; DC, dichorionic; MA, monoamniotic; DA, diamniotic; TTT, twin–twin transfusion

Table 2.2 Ultrasound determination of chorionicity and amnionicity

Septum	Thick	Thin	None	Total
Placentation (pathology)				
DC	420	14	6	440
MC, DA	17	110	17	144
MC, MA	0	0	12	12
Total	437	124	35	596

DC, dichorionic; MC, monochorionic; DA, diamniotic; MA, monoamniotic

Data based on ten published series, not analyzed by gestational age at time of ultrasound diagnosis

merely for the detection of DC twins or to report septal membrane thickness as 'indeterminate', but to delineate the high-risk MC pregnancies from all others. *Septal membrane thickness is the criterion even if it is discordant with the number of placental disks.* The underdiagnosis of MC twins may have serious consequences later in the pregnancy (Table 2.1; see also Part III, *Impact of chorionicity on the lives of twins*). Collation from the published literature of the results of ultrasound diagnosis of chorionicity reflects the sensitivity and specificity of this modality (Table 2.2). The main concern raised by these data is the 17 (12%) MC cases that were 'underdiagnosed' as DC. The 'overdiagnosis' of DC cases as MC (and therefore at higher risk) is not a clinical problem.

In summary, the advantages of first-trimester ultrasound examinations in twin pregnancies are:

(1) In DC twins, the chorions are more likely to be seen as clearly separate because fusion and thinning occurs with later growth;

(2) If the twins are MC and develop TTT, the membranes are less distinct later when hydramnios / oligohydramnios is present;

(3) MC twins can be more expeditiously assessed with ultrasound for growth discordance and development of polyhydramnios / oligohydramnios, with an opportunity for early treatment of antepartum TTT; and

(4) Rapid decisions can later be taken in cases of impending fetal death on the basis of the earlier obtained certain knowledge of chorionicity.

Number of embryos

The distinction between twin pregnancies and HOMPs is important because of the even higher risks of premature labor in the latter compared with the former. Several clinical errors may occur:

(1) Artefactual reflections may lead to over-diagnosis of the embryo number;

(2) Third, fourth and fifth embryos may not be diagnosed initially;

(3) Spontaneous reductions may occur, with the 'vanishing twin' phenomenon being manifested between successive ultrasound examinations;

(4) The number of embryos detected by ultrasound may exceed the number of zygotes implanted, as MZ twins are two-and-one-half times more common in ART than in spontaneous twin pregnancies and HOMPs; and

(5) Bewildering combinations of (3) and (4) may occur (Figure 2.4, page 116).

In clinical practice, the sonographer should not stop after encountering the same number of gestations as the number of implanted embryos. Repeat ultrasound is mandatory as pregnancy progresses to allow diagnosis of the true number of embryos and to document MC twinning and / or spontaneous resorption, if either of these events should occur.

Doppler studies

Doppler studies assess placental vascular resistance using the umbilical arterial pulsatility index (PI). This may be useful in singleton and multiple pregnancies with intrauterine growth retardation.

Because MC twins often have placental vascular connections, additional complexities in umbilical flow measurement may be present. With TTT, there are no functional superficial vascular anastomoses, and increased placental resistance is present in both the donor and the recipient twin. In contrast, no differences in PI are seen in MC twins that are discordant for growth, but with no evidence of TTT. Thus, a PI that falls outside the normal range is probably a predictor of the onset of hydrops in the recipient, and may be an indication for active intervention.

Doppler flow studies can assess the results of therapeutic amniocentesis and evaluate regional blood flow patterns in the twin fetuses. In general, venous flow is reduced in both the donors and recipients, and pulsatile venous flow may be seen in the recipients. There is usually a reduced blood flow in the aorta and major arteries in both donors and recipients before treatment of TTT. A variety of changes in arterial blood flow may occur subsequent to therapeutic amniocentesis, presumably reflecting the physiological responses to the various alterations, such as those in placental function or blood gas status. Many recipients develop tricuspid regurgitation, and dilatation of the inferior vena cava, ductus venosus, hepatic and umbilical veins, with transmission of pulsatile flow.

Doppler studies are also useful in mapping the anatomy of fetal vessels on the placental surface and in looking for abnormal flow patterns. Such studies may in future delineate the vessels involved in the a→v anastomoses of prenatal chronic TTT. Doppler assessment of the pulsatile flow direction can identify the cords of pump and acardiac twins in TRAP. The diagnosis of entwined cords of MA, MC twins is facilitated by Doppler flow studies (see below). Finally, Doppler studies can document dramatic dynamic reverses in blood flow when the donor TTT / MC twin dies. These changes probably cause the acute hypotension / hypoxia / anemia in the surviving recipient leading to organ necrosis.

Vanishing twins

One published analysis estimates that as many as ten times the number of twins are conceived as are born. The excess revert to singleton status in the late first or early second trimester through the phenomenon of 'vanishing', a term which simply describes the process of natural resorption. Serial ultrasound examinations can confirm this diagnosis if the loss occurs after clinical pregnancy is established.

Twins may vanish both in naturally conceived multiple pregnancies and in those resulting from ART. In this latter instance, however, the rate of MZ twins is increased by approximately three times that of normal. Thus, although a known number of embryos may be implanted by IVF, any combination of MZ splitting and vanishing may subsequently modify the number.

Fetal death of one twin

With DC twins, the death of one fetus usually has no adverse effects on the co-twin and, in clinical practice, the dead DC fetus is often left *in utero* to be delivered (as a stillborn or a fetus papyraceus) with the survivor at a later date. Alternatively, the dead fetus may spontaneously deliver separately, following which the surviving twin may continue *in utero* for several weeks, certainly up to, and often past, the stage of pulmonary maturity.

If the twins are MC, the death of one of them in the second or third trimester can have major consequences for the survivor. The antepartum demise of one MC twin is usually the result of placental vascular disease – either TTT or TRAP – and may occur despite optimal management. In contrast to DC twins, the consequences for the MC co-twin survivor are often severe, most likely as a result of the rapid changes in arterial blood flow and pressure in the single placenta leading to visceral shut-down and / or organ infarction.

In the second trimester, infarction may involve the intestine and skin (widespread aplasia cutis) whereas, in the third trimester, the brain (Figure 2.5, page 117), kidneys, liver and lungs are more likely to be affected. These latter changes occur shortly after the death of the affected twin, as documented by fortuitously timed ultrasound studies.

Given these considerations, even emergency delivery may not preclude organ damage to the survivor once the co-twin has died. Indeed, it is debatable whether imminent fetal death can always be adequately predicted so as to permit preventive delivery of the expected survivor, especially in the face of the risks of complications for preterm delivery.

Complications of monochorionic twin pregnancy

Twin–twin transfusion (TTT)

The most important complication of MC twin pregnancy is chronic antenatal TTT. Paradoxically, there are no universally agreed-upon criteria for the antenatal diagnosis of TTT. There are two primary reasons for this:

(1) Growth discrepancy *per se* (often a feature of TTT) is not always indicative of TTT, but may be the result of unequal placental sharing. Moreover, not all TTT twins are growth-discordant; and

(2) Anemia, hydrops and hydramnios in twin pregnancy (including MC twins) may have causes other than TTT.

In spite of these apparent drawbacks, it is possible to develop a working plan for the antenatal diagnosis for TTT which includes:

(1) Definitive diagnosis of MC twins (whether DA or MA);

(2) Oligohydramnios / hydramnios, with the presence of a 'stuck' oliguric twin in MC, DA (but not MC, MA) twins (Figure 2.6 a, page 117);

(3) Kidneys and urinary bladder that are small in the donor and large in the recipient;

(4) Discordance in sizes of fetal hearts, livers and umbilical cords (Figure 2.6 b & c, page 118)

when / if the recipient develops cardiac decompensation. Right ventricular hypertrophy, tricuspid regurgitation causing dilatation and abnormal blood flow in the inferior vena cava (Figure 2.6 d & e, page 119), ductus venosus (Figure 2.7 a & b, page 120), hepatic veins and umbilical vein of the recipient, and abnormal systemic arterial waveforms may also be seen (Figure 2.7 c & d, pages 121–2);

(5) Rapid reaccumulation of amniotic fluid in the recipient's sac after therapeutic amniocentesis; biophysical response of the donor to amniocentesis with amniotic fluid production and fetal growth;

(6) Fetal growth discordance (not always present; Figure 2.7 e, page 122);

(7) Discordant hematocrit and plasma protein levels by umbilical blood sampling (not always present);

(8) Temporary paralysis of both twins after intravascular infusion of pancuronium into the cord of one twin;

(9) Transfer of injected adult red cells from donor to recipient;

(10) Fetal serum erythropoietin levels (elevated in both twins in the presence of TTT, but only in the smaller twin when growth discordance is due to other factors); and

(11) Elevated atrial natriuretic factor in the recipient twin.

Given that the diagnosis of fully developed antenatal TTT can be made using the diagnostic criteria noted above, it remains to be seen whether this diagnosis can be made in its earliest stages and, if so, whether earlier compared with later treatment always yields better results. (Examples of the early diagnosis and treatment of TTT are shown in Part III.) No substantial progress can be made in this area of obstetrics until all MC twin pregnancies are reliably diagnosed in the first trimester and then carefully followed-up so that the natural history of the initiating events of TTT is better understood.

Twin reversed arterial perfusion (TRAP)

The diagnosis of TRAP can be difficult if the ultrasonographer is not familiar with the entity (Figure 2.7 f, page 122). The acardiac fetus may be mistaken for a fibroid or a malformed and dead fetus. The most common diagnosis is that of a dead anencephalic fetus but, even then, appearances can be misleading as spinal reflexes may remain intact. In such a circumstance, the apparently 'dead' fetus has been observed to kick actively rather than be moved passively by the pump twin.

Reversed umbilical arterial blood flow towards the acardiac fetus can be documented by Doppler examination. Doppler is also capable of assessing the umbilical arterial PI as well as the arterial and venous flows within the fetuses themselves.

Acardiac fetuses usually have a single umbilical artery (Figure 2.8 a, page 123). The passive nature of the blood flow in the acardiac fetal cord may be apparent through fluctuations caused by respiratory activity of the pump twin (see Figure 2.8 a). Large communicating vessels may be seen running from the cord of the acardiac twin out onto the chorionic surface of the placenta (Figure 2.8 b, page 123).

Monoamniotic twins

Diagnosis of MC, MA twin pregnancy by the absence of separating septal membranes should prompt an immediate search for entangled cords (Figure 2.9 a–d, pages 124–5). With or without entangled cords, MA twins are still at risk not only for TTT (Figure 2.9 e, page 126) and TRAP, but also for intrapartum cord complications (Figures 2.10 and 2.11, pages 126–7).

Conjoined twins

Conjoined twins (Figure 2.12, page 127) are most often MC, MA and can be diagnosed by observation of a constant relationship between the twin body axes. Depending on the stage of pregnancy at the time of diagnosis, the therapeutic options include pregnancy termination, postpartum surgical separation or no intervention. Conjoined twins that are not separable include cephalothoracopagus, dicephalus and diprosopus twins (see Section 3, *Conjoined twinning*).

Congenital anomalies

Congenital anomalies are probably more common in MZ twins than in DZ twins and singletons. The extent of these differences is not always clear and may reflect ascertainment biases in data collection. Apart from anomalies intrinsic to MC, MZ twins (for example, acardius or conjoined twins), a wide range of true malformations is seen (see Section 3, *Discordance for congenital anomalies in MZ twins*).

Published reports indicate that midline malformations, such as neural-tube defects, omphalocele, cloacal exstrophy (Figure 2.13, page 128) and congenital heart disease, are most commonly seen in MZ twins. *It is important to recall that MZ twins concordant for major malformations are rare. It is wrong to assume that twins discordant for malformation are always DZ (and hence DC).* If a fatal malformation is found in one twin, selective termination is an option, provided that the twins are DC (regardless of zygosity) and that such a procedure is technically feasible. In contrast, it is unwise to attempt 'selective' termination in MC twins unless the methods to be used involve total isolation of the two circulations, as they are likely to be in communication via placental vascular anastomoses.

There have been reports in the literature of cases in which a malformed fetus, presumed to be a DC twin, was given either an intracardiac injection of potassium chloride or an air embolism, which then also resulted in the death of the normal MC co-twin shortly thereafter. Such events may be presumed to be caused by the agent reaching the normal co-twin via a shared circulation or by the major changes in cardiovascular dynamics following immediately upon death of the malformed twin and transmitted to the co-twin via anastomoses in the MC placenta.

Prenatal diagnosis of genetic disease: Amniocentesis, and chorionic villus and umbilical blood sampling

These procedures are generally safe to carry out in twin pregnancies. With DC twins, samples can reliably be collected from each twin (Figure 2.14, page 128). With those MC twins who have different chromosomal constitutions, it is not yet clear whether both cell lines are likely to be expressed in the chorionic villi. However, it is probable that the amniotic fluid of MC, DA twins reflects the chromosomal constitutions of the relevant twin. Techniques have been described in which the two amniotic fluid samples are collected with only one pass of the needle by advancing it across the septum to collect the second sample. However, this is not without the possibility of causing a major septal tear, thereby converting the pregnancy from MC, DA to pseudo-MC, MA with all the attendant risks of cord complications.

Congenital anomalies that cause elevated amniotic fluid AFP may cause confusion in MC, DA twins. In these circumstances, the septum may be so thin that AFP from the affected twin is able to diffuse into the sac of the other twin. The result is not only a false-positive, but may potentially lead to the erroneous conclusion that both twins are malformed. Fetal death of one MC twin can also cause a raised AFP in the sac of the co-twin, leading to extensive investigation for anomalies associated with an elevated level of AFP. This problem may also arise after selective fetal reduction. Such considerations do not apply to DC twins.

There is no point in sampling umbilical blood from both twins for genetic diseases if they are MC because the presence of vascular anastomoses will almost certainly contaminate the samples. In addition, discordance for single-gene diseases on a simple Mendelian basis has not yet been convincingly demonstrated in MZ twin pairs.

Antenatal zygosity testing

On rare occasions, indications for prenatal zygosity testing may be present. If chorionicity has not been determined in early pregnancy, the impending fetal death of one twin of a like-sexed pair poses a particular problem. If the twins are DC (regardless of zygosity), it may be safe to allow the pregnancy to continue. Unfortunately, it may be impossible to make a reliable determinion of chorionicity in the second and third trimesters. It may then be helpful to test zygosity by DNA restriction fragment length polymorphism (RFLP) analysis of amniotic fluid cells from each fetus (see Part II, Section 2). If the twins are DZ, they must be DC whereas, if they are MZ, they may be either MC or DC.

Selective termination

This procedure may be indicated for a severe congenital anomaly in one twin or for vascular complications in MC twins, such as antenatal TTT and TRAP. It should not be assumed that twins discordant for major congenital anomalies are necessarily DZ. Indeed, in cases where one MZ

twin is malformed, the co-twin may be less severely affected with the same disease or even completely unaffected.

Selective termination using standard methods is relatively safe in DC twins. However, these standard methods should not be used in MC twins. In such cases, the circulation of the affected fetus needs to be completely isolated from that of the twin to be conserved. Therapeutic modalities remain experimental at present, and include selective delivery of the fetus via hysterotomy and ligation or clipping of the umbilical cord.

Antenatal surgery in twin pregnancy

The presence of twins increases the compexity of the indications, techniques and sequelae of fetal surgery. Surgical intervention may be indicated for intrinsic complications of MC twinning itself (TTT and TRAP). The twins may be discordant for a potentially correctable anomaly, but the operation itself may place the unaffected twin at unacceptable risk. Therefore, individual cases should be managed with consideration of the given merits. The underlying consideration is that MC twins are much less likely than DC twins to tolerate surgical procedures without developing complications.

Antenatal diagnosis of higher-order multiple pregnancy (HOMP)

The survival of HOMPs is inversely proportional to the number of fetuses present mostly because the frequency of markedly preterm delivery increases with the number of fetuses.

Naturally conceived HOMPs differ biologically from those induced by ART. Spontaneous HOMPs include large proportions of MZ fetuses, many of which are also MC and therefore at risk for vascular complications. In contrast, approximately 10% of ART-induced HOMPs comprise MZ fetuses as well as combinations of MZ and DZ twins. This suggests that multiple ART zygotes may split on occasions to give rise to even higher-order HOMPs than were originally anticipated.

Thus, it is incorrect to assume that the final number of embryos visualized by the fifth week of gestation corresponds directly with the number of zygotes originally inserted into the uterus. Unusual combinations of MZ twinning and vanishing twins can occur in ART-induced as well as spontaneous HOMPs (see Figure 2.4). Figure 2.15a (page 129) shows naturally conceived trichorionic (TC) triplets who proved at birth to be MZ. Figure 2.15b & c (page 129) shows septachorionic septuplets conceived by induced ovulation. Selective termination was eventually performed.

Assessment of fetal wellbeing

Standard methods are used to assess the wellbeing of both twins. Growth rates are generally assessed by ultrasonography. Although charts for antenatal twin growth are available, most clinicians recognize that, up to 32 weeks, twin growth is similar to singleton growth. As yet, there is no agreement as to when the growth process deviates; various studies have cited a range of 32–35 weeks. Growth discordance is frequent in DZ and MZ twins, and may be problematical for their diagnosis and management.

Further improvements in ultrasound examination

Key advances may soon occur in the early diagnosis and management of TTT. Agreement needs to be reached about criteria for the earliest possible diagnosis of TTT as well as the earliest time at which interventions may be planned. Early treatment may reduce complication rates and improve the proportion of TTT fetuses who survive intact. Crucial diagnostic features could include: growth discordance; hydramnios / oligohydramnios; and velamentous cord insertion of the donor. Ultrasound may also be able to map the types of anastomoses in the chorionic plate. Artery-to-artery ($a \leftrightarrow a$) connections have been documented by ultrasound. If uncompensated arteriovenous ($a \rightarrow v$) anastomoses can be found, they are diagnostic of TTT. In the event that laser coagulation were to become the treatment of choice, knowledge of the precise location of the $a \rightarrow v$ anastomosis might permit rapid and specific coagulation.

Summary

Among the many ways in which ultrasonography is useful in the management of twin pregnancy, *none is more important than the determination of chorionicity.* This can be most reliably determined by ultrasound in the first trimester. The accurate assessment of chorionicity offers obstetricians an opportunity to manage MC twins more intensively and expectantly than is required for DC twins. MC twins behave in unpredictable ways that result in high rates of mortality and morbidity for both fetuses. It appears reasonable to expect that these rates will be reduced if MC twins are diagnosed and actively managed from the earliest time of onset of complications long before any symptoms arise (see Part I, Section 3).

Section 3 Understanding the pathology of twin pregnancies

Introduction

Twin pregnancies carry high risks for both the mother and her fetuses. The maternal and fetal expression of these risks varies enormously, and it is inadvisable to extrapolate statistical frequencies to individual cases. These risks may become apparent in the ante-, intra- or postpartum periods, and are generally specific to each stage of pregnancy.

Risks in the antepartum period include increased likelihood of fetal death and maternal bleeding, preterm labor and delivery, hydramnios, anemia and pregnancy-induced hypertension. A unique set of risks (not present in other subsets of twins) is seen in MC twin pairs during the second and third trimesters because of the frequent presence of placental vascular communication.

Intrapartum problems include delivery of undiagnosed twins, malpresentations, cord prolapse and other cord complications, and locked twins. Postpartum maternal difficulties include an increased risk of hemorrhage from acute and delayed uterine atony and, possibly, depression.

Neonatal considerations are centered on short- and longterm complications of preterm delivery, management of sequelae of placental vascular anastomoses, diagnosis and management of congenital malformations, and recognition and treatment of complications caused by asphyxia / hypoxia / hypotension, low birth weight and / or intrauterine growth retardation.

Statistics of morbidity and mortality

Perinatal mortality rates associated with both singleton and multiple pregnancies have fallen markedly over the past 20 years. However, perinatal mortality remains three to four times higher for multifetal compared with singleton pregnancies, despite vast improvements in obstetric and newborn medicine. This greater mortality is due in part to the increased background risks for pregnancy-induced hypertension and antepartum hemorrhage, and to the intrinsic problems associated with MC twin pregnancies because of their vascular complications (see Table 1.2).

Although fetal and neonatal deaths in DC twins are often unpredictable (maternal pregnancy-induced hypertension and / or antepartum hemorrhage) or unpreventable (lethal malformation), they are usually single and the co-twin often survives. In contrast, with MC twinning, it is common for both twins to die or for the survivor to suffer severe sequelae of the death of the co-twin. These sequelae are mediated via the interfetal vascular anastomoses and sharing of the single (MC) placenta.

The morbidity and mortality rates for twins (and HOMPs) are both greatly influenced by the enormous (tenfold) differential in the frequency of preterm (< 37 weeks) and extremely preterm (< 32 weeks) deliveries, and low (< 2500 g) and dangerously low (< 1500 g) birthweights of twins compared with singletons. Moreover, the occurrence of major malformations may be more common in MZ twins than in DZ twins or singletons, and is a further cause of morbidity and mortality.

Preterm labor and delivery

Why twin pregnancies are predisposed to preterm labor and delivery has not been fully elucidated. An element of this predisposition may relate to the background medical circumstances, such as hypertensive disorders of pregnancy, management of fetal death, abruption, placenta previa and serious complications of MC placentation, which may lead to immediate plans for delivery, although it is recognized that the fetus will be preterm.

In the majority of cases, no specific event triggers early delivery, and the mother spontaneously begins labor for reasons that remain unclear. The bulk of the gestational contents (at all gestational ages) is frequently cited as a prime factor initiating a pentad of events that begins with premature cervical dilatation, increased uterine muscular irritability, early labor, ruptured membranes and, possibly, ascending infection as a culminating feature.

As far as the authors are aware, the specific contribution of various factors leading to preterm labor and delivery have not been quantified. In view of these uncertainties and in the absence of truly effective methods to halt all instances of preterm labor, a reasonable commonsense approach would be to avoid those circumstances that are widely believed to predispose to it. Among the most frequently cited predisposing factors is strenuous physical activity. As a precaution, activity restrictions should begin shortly after 20 weeks, supplemented by early maternity leave for mothers who work outside the home.

Specific problems and complications of monochorionic twin pregnancy

There are problems specific to MC twins that account for the especially high risks and the need for more intensive antenatal monitoring. Although numerous authorities claim that the frequency of major malformations is higher in MZ than in either DZ twins or singletons, the literature on congenital malformations in twins provides scant documentary evidence on the chorionicity of malformed MZ twins. A small minority (around 5%) of MC twins are also MA, a condition which puts them at further risk for cord complications. Conjoined twins are, by definition, MC and are usually MA.

A small but unquantified number of MC twins have complications as a result of the vascular anatomy of their placentas, including TTT (both pre- and perinatal), TRAP, unequally shared perfusion of the placental parenchyma, damage to the survivor when one fetus dies and complications due to attempts at selective termination. These complications are best understood in the context of the unique vascular connections found in MC placentas. The precise frequency of these complications among MC twins is not known, and estimates vary widely. According to the more commonly quoted figures, TTT ('stuck twin' or oligohydramnios) occurs in 20–30% of MC twins and TRAP in 1%.

Anatomy of monochorionic twin placentas

The optimal management of complications in twin pregnancies cannot be carried out if the chorionicity is unknown. With DC placentas, regardless of whether the disks are separate or fused, the chorionic component of the septum usually forms a virtually impermeable barrier to effectively segregate the two fetal circulations (Figures 3.1 and 3.2, page 130). It therefore follows that any adverse biophysical event in one DC twin, such as growth retardation or fetal death, can be ascribed to specific factors operating only in the relevant twin's feto-placental unit with a minimal effect, if any, on the health of the co-twin. Should it be desirable to continue a pregnancy to allow a surviving DC twin to achieve pulmonary maturation after the death of its co-twin in the second trimester, this should be possible with relative safety. In rare instances, selective delivery of the deceased twin fetus may be feasible.

The situation with MC twins is in stark contrast to the one described above because there usually are subtle and complex relationships between the circulations of the twin pair (see Figure 3.1) which cause the biophysical status of one twin to affect that of the other.

The vascular relationships in the MC placenta are based upon two principles:

(1) Anastomotic connections of various types and combinations are present in around 90% of MC placentas (Figure 3.3 a, page 131). These anastomoses arise because the MC placenta is a truly single (not fused) organ, and the anatomical distribution of the fetal vessels running to and from the two umbilical cords is not limited by a septal chorionic component. Only around 10% of MC placentas have no anastomoses (Figure 3.3 b, page 131).

The placental blood vessels develop separately from those of the embryo proper so that the two fully formed parenchymal systems come to meet near the body stalk (Figure 3.3 c, page 132). In a given MC twin placenta, there is an infinite number of ways in which the primary placental circulation may be linked to the two twin circulations (see Figure 3.3 c). Indeed, *the whole of the parenchyma of an MC placenta is potentially available for perfusion by either or both twins, just as the whole parenchyma of a singleton gestation is available to the singleton fetus.* Each MC placenta has a unique vascular anatomical configuration; however, certain general patterns are commonly observed (see below).

(2) The intuitive expectation that a single placental disk would be shared equally is incorrect. As a result of the unpredictable and virtually random vascular 'commitments' of placental parenchymal perfusion zones to each twin, significantly unequal sharing of parenchymal mass and function is common because of differences in the sizes of the arterial and venous fields of each twin (Figure 3.4, page 133). Patterns of cord insertions largely determine the degree of unequal sharing.

Unfortunately, the MC twin placental structure originates from one zygote and receives developmental instructions to function as a singleton placenta. Thus, the failure of the MC placenta to appreciate that it serves two masters and must keep their circulations separate is a 'fatal flaw' of its physiology. It is this flaw that leads to the particular patterns of anastomoses and sharing described below. In turn, these patterns largely determine the number of adverse clinical outcomes in which the biophysical status of one twin has a definite impact on that of the co-twin, leading to an increased (double) morbidity and mortality.

Because the anatomy of each MC placenta is unique, the clinical behavior and development of complications in MC twins is unpredictable. Some of the presently experimental methods to treat these complications involve the deliberate segregation of the two fetal circulations. Indeed, no MC twins are 'safe' until they are disconnected from their placenta (and thereby from each other).

On rare occasions, instead of the typical single-disked MC placenta (see Figures 3.3 and 3.4), the disk is divided into two separate masses that are either connected by a narrow bridge of parenchyma (Figure 3.5 a, page 134) or remain completely separate (Figure 3.5 b, page 134), as with bilobar singleton placentas. These appearances may cause confusion in the antenatal diagnosis of chorionicity as two disks are apparently seen, albeit with a thin septum. The bilobar MC placenta is likely to function similarly to a DC placenta as few, if any, significant anastomoses are present between the lobes.

The two unique vascular characteristics of MC placentas (presence of anastomoses and unequal parenchymal sharing) may occur alone or in combination, and are often causally linked (Figure 3.6, page 135). Their net effect is a considerable sharing and / or overlap of the two circulations, rendering it difficult to assign the perfusion zones of particular arteries and veins to a specific twin. These complexities may also result in a number of adverse hemodynamic events that account for most, but not all, of the greater frequency of perinatal morbidity and mortality in MC, compared with DC, twins.

Careful study of the vascular anatomy of MC placentas after delivery permits a better understanding of the mechanisms underlying the differing severity and nature of these adverse events, as well as their appropriate antenatal diagnosis and management in other pregnancies on the basis of antenatal assessment and inference of presumed vascular anatomy.

The anastomotic vessels of MC placentas are either superficial or deep (see Figure 1.12). Superficial anastomoses are functionally bidirectional or reversible (except in TRAP pairs), and run directly in the potential space between the chorionic plate and the amnion. They may connect arteries to arteries (a↔a; see Figures 3.3a and 3.4a&b) or veins to veins (v↔v). The a↔a connections are far more common than the v↔v connections.

In contrast, arteriovenous (a→v) anastomoses are always deep and unidirectional. They do not lie on the placental surface, but rather are only found deep in the parenchyma, where zones of arterial perfusion by one twin overlap zones of venous collection by the co-twin (see Figures 3.3a and 3.4a). These connections are usually due to the disproportion between the sizes of the arterial and venous zones of a given twin (and hence between the sizes of the venous and arterial zones of the co-twin). On the surface, these zones are identified by the appearance of an artery from one twin dipping down through a foramen from the chorionic plate into the parenchyma, at a point where the corresponding vein from that perfusion unit emerges onto the chorionic plate, before connecting up with the umbilical venous system of the co-twin. Thus, the two vessels appear to be 'nose-to-nose' (Figure 3.7a, page 136). NO DIRECT A→V CONNECTIONS ARE EVER SEEN ON THE SURFACE.

Variations in the presence / absence / combination of vascular anastomoses together with the varying degrees of unequal parenchymal sharing result in the complex array of clinical outcomes seen in MC twins, including:

(1) Uncomplicated delivery close to term without growth discordance or other complications due to: (a) bilobar MC disk (see Figure 3.5), (b) equal vascular sharing without anastomoses (see Figure 3.3b) or (c) equal vascular sharing with superficial anastomoses, among other possibilities;

(2) Marked growth discordance without TTT caused by: (a) unequal parenchymal sharing without anastomoses or (b) unequal parenchymal sharing with superficial anastomoses, with or without a→v anastomoses (see Figure 3.4);

(3) Severe antenatal TTT, which usually occurs when an a→v anastomosis is not compensated by functional a↔a or v↔v superficial anastomoses (see below, *Mechanisms of twin–twin transfusion*);

(4) Acute perinatal transfusion, wherein large volumes of blood are rapidly transfused via a↔a and / or v↔v anastomoses. Similar routes are used when one MC fetus dies and the co-twin develops acute hypotension (see below, *Mechanisms of twin–twin transfusion*); and

(5) TRAP, wherein large, direct, unidirectional a→a and v→v anastomoses connect the pump twin with the acardiac fetus (see below, *Mechanisms of acardius*).

As both the a↔a and a→v connections are frequent findings, both are often present in combination in MC placentas. In these cases, the most common arrangement (see Figures 3.3a and 3.4) is such that any significant volume of blood transfused via the a→v connection is returned from the recipient to the donor via the a↔a anastomosis as soon as there is a difference in arterial blood pressure between the twins (see Figure 3.7e, page 137). Thus, the a↔a anastomosis serves as an 'overflow' or 'safety' valve. When only a↔a anastomoses are present, there is usually little, if any, net flow as long as both twins have similar biophysical status.

In contrast to a↔a and a→v anastomoses, v↔v connections are rare, whether alone or in combination. Such connections are often associated with poor outcomes, possibly because large volumes of blood are rapidly transferred in the low-pressure venous system. Rates of v↔v flow may also be markedly affected by changes in intra-amniotic cavity pressure. Indeed, v↔v flow may be intermittent.

The 'reopening' of v↔v connections is most likely one of the mechanisms whereby serial amniocentesis is sometimes successful in reversing severe antepartum TTT. IT IS THE PRESENCE OF DEEP A→V ANASTOMOSIS ALONE, UNCOMPENSATED BY FUNCTIONAL SUPERFICIAL ANASTOMOSES OF EITHER VARIETY, THAT MOST OFTEN CAUSES ANTENATAL TTT WITH ITS ADVERSE OUTCOMES.

Mechanisms of twin–twin transfusion

Chronic antepartum transfusion

If an a→v anastomosis is the sole vascular connection, the twins are locked into a chronic prenatal donor/recipient relationship that is characterized by uncompensated transfusion of blood from one twin to the other, resulting in antenatal TTT (see Figure 3.7). The a→v anastomosis of an MC placenta is the only known naturally occurring (non-pathological) structure that can bring about the death of two human beings on a predictable basis.

Just as there is no consensus on criteria for the diagnosis of prenatal TTT (see Part I, Section 2, *Complications of monochorionic twin pregnancy*), there is scant information as to the volume of

transfused blood required to initiate the syndrome. The anatomy of the anastomoses seen in the placenta at birth may not accurately reflect the situation *in vivo* at the onset of prenatal TTT. Much remains to be learned before anatomically precise and effective methods can be used to treat TTT.

Once an antepartum episode of whole blood transfusion begins, which may be sudden and of significant volume, a complex cascade of events ensues (Figure 3.8, page 138; see also Table 3.1). The donor may enter a phase of peripheral vascular shutdown which results in renal hypoperfusion and oliguria.

Because the donor has had a smaller venous share of the placenta, preexisting nutritional deprivation may possibly predispose to hypertension, transfusion across the a→v anastomosis and visceral (including renal) hypofunction. Oliguria leads to oligohydramnios and, unless placentation is MA, the twin becomes 'stuck' in its own sac.

In addition, the donor's plasma may become hypoosmolar due to protein loss through the blood transfusion, thereby possibly causing water to pass into the maternal circulation and 'drying out' the fetus, thus exacerbating growth delay and oligohydramnios.

Growth lag may result from the decreased peripheral circulation as well as the smaller share of placental venous return (see above). Erythropoietin levels in the donor rise, although the anemia may not be of long duration. However, erythropoietin from the donor may reach the recipient if further or ongoing transfusion occurs, thus exacerbating the red-cell overload of the recipient. However, there may be little difference between the red-cell counts and hematocrits of the donor and recipient. It has been suggested that, because of its malnourished state, the donor may synthesize growth factors which may also be transfused to the recipient, thereby exacerbating growth discordance.

Responses of the recipient to hypervolemia from the transfused blood are atrial dilatation, atriopeptin secretion and polyuria, all resulting in hydramnios. The recipient's kidneys are able to ultrafiltrate low-molecular-weight plasma proteins, electrolytes and water, but are unable to unload plasma proteins of high molecular weight or blood cells. Hyperosmolality, hyperviscosity and elevated hematocrit develop. (The situation can be likened to a salt pan to which saltwater is being added, but from which only water vapor can evaporate.) Overall, the osmolarity of the twin and its amniotic fluid increases, and maternal water is probably recruited in the production of hypervolemia and hydramnios.

Because of the hyperviscosity, increased peripheral resistance to predominantly right ventricular cardiac output leads to compensatory cardiac hypertrophy; if this hypertrophy is inadequate for maintaining cardiac output, cardiac failure follows, ultimately resulting in hydrops and fetal death. Arrhythmias may supervene. Recipients with right ventricular hypertrophy who survive the fetal period often have persistent cardiomyopathy which may eventually prove fatal. There may be sufficient tricuspid incompetence and stasis to cause stenosis or atresia of the ductus venosus. Temporary tricuspid valvular stenosis has also been described in a donor twin.

It is not clear whether the donor or recipient is at greater risk for fetal death, but most authors believe it is the recipient who is in greater danger. Attempts at selective rescue are therefore usually directed towards saving the donor. A small number of cases of TTT resolve spontaneously; others improve after the death of one twin. In general, however, the rate of mortality for both twins is high without interventional management.

Among the more recently described treatments for prenatal TTT is amniocentesis of the recipient sac, which often requires serial removal of one or more litres of amniotic fluid. This intervention may result in improvement of the biophysical status of both fetuses (Table 3.1), but the mechanism(s) underlying improvement remain obscure. One possible explanation is that small $v \leftrightarrow v$ anastomoses may be present in addition to the $a \rightarrow v$ connection. Five mechanisms may cause such connections to cease function as TTT develops:

(1) Because of hyperviscosity, $v \leftrightarrow v$ flow may cease after the original TTT event;

(2) Onset of increased intra-amniotic pressure in the recipient's sac may further reduce flow in the low-pressure thin-walled veins, and amniocentesis may sufficiently relieve the pressure in the amniotic cavity to allow these $v \leftrightarrow v$ connections to function again, with compensatory return of blood from recipient to donor;

(3) The umbilical cord is velamentously inserted into the septum in some cases of TTT. When hydramnios develops, the base of the diamniotic septum tends to shift, stretching the fetal vessels

Table 3.1 Results of large-volume amniocentesis for treatment of antepartum twin–twin transfusion

	Fetuses	Survivors	% Survivors
With amniocentesis	268	164	57
Without amniocentesis	90	34	38*

Data are based on 17 series published from 1985 onwards. There is no analysis by gestational age, presence/absence of hydrops, presence/absence of established labor at time of clinical presentation or long-term follow-up studies of survivors for rates of morbidity

*Rate with conservative management; this suggests that the prognosis is not as poor as usually reported

as they leave the septum to run onto the chorionic plate (Figure 3.9 a, page 139). The effects of such stretching are likely to be more severe on thin-walled low-pressure veins, and can be reversed by amniocentesis. Having said this, both cords are normally inserted into the disk in the majority of MC placentas. Thus, if the septum moves because of increased pressure in one sac, the pressure may then be transmitted to v↔v anastomoses (Figure 3.9 b, page 139) and may also have a 'pruning' effect on peripheral venous branches of the donor twin, thereby further worsening the biophysical status of that fetus;

(4) Improvement in urine production by the donor may be brought about by relief of the amniotic fluid pressure on the chorionic plate veins near the septum; and

(5) Tricuspid incompetence and reflux into the umbilical vein may be sufficient to prevent flow in v↔v anastomoses. Certainly, it has been observed that the placenta may appear to be flattened and attenuated prior to amniocentesis, only returning to its normal plump shape afterwards.

A different albeit experimental approach to treatment involves segregation of the circulations of the twins by deliberate vascular occlusion. At present, this is achieved by laser coagulation of the vessels running to and from the placental equatorial zone. The approach is made from the sac of the recipient.

It is hoped that clinically useful methods (such as Doppler flow studies) will soon be found to select specific vessels for coagulation (as, for example, it is clear that only veins are involved on the recipient side of the a→v anastomosis). It should be borne in mind that the artery and vein involved in an a→v anastomosis are 'nose-to-nose' on the chorionic surface, and should be readily identifiable.

Table 3.2 Results of laser surgery for twin–twin transfusion

Reference	Cases (n)	Gestational age (GA)* (weeks)	Gain in GA (weeks)	Survivors (n / %)
De Lia et al., 1995	26	18–24 (21)**	6–17 (12)**	28 / 53† (53%)**
Ville et al., 1995	45	15–28 (21)**	0–21 (14)**	45 / 90†† (50%)**

*At diagnosis or time of procedure;

†Includes one set of triplets, and one survivor who has neurological impairment;

††25% of survivors have neurological impairment;

**Median

Non-selective coagulation of all vessels at the equatorial zone may possibly reduce placental arterial perfusion of one or both twins, and the donor may already be marginally nourished. However, global vessel coagulation should protect the survivor if the other twin dies *in utero*. Although the number of patients receiving this form of management is thus far small, results are at least comparable with those of serial amniocentesis (Figures 3.9 c & d, page 140; Table 3.2). It appears that, the earlier in gestation the procedure is performed, the greater the prolongation of pregnancy. This may be a reflection of early diagnosis before the disease process has run its course.

Selective termination of the more seriously affected twin has been advocated to preserve the life of the other. Inadvertent (and uncontrolled) loss of significant blood volume during cordocentesis can also relieve the effects of TTT.

Septostomy of the dividing membranes has recently been reported to reverse antepartum TTT. The mechanism is unclear.

Acute intrapartum transfusion

Chronic antepartum transfusional events should not be confused with acute intrapartum TTT, which may occur *de novo* in the absence of antepartum TTT, or as a confusing and confounding event following antepartum TTT (Figure 3.10 a–d, page 141). Because of the connections between the circulations of MC twins, cord clamping after the delivery of the first twin immediately affects the relationship of the unborn twin to the entire placental parenchyma until that second twin is delivered.

In such circumstances, at least two sequelae, each with opposite results, are possible:

(1) The sudden elimination of arterial perfusion by the first-born twin may create, in the second twin, new hypotensive areas of placental perfusion with acute volume loss; or

(2) More commonly, a residue of blood in the mutual placental parenchyma is suddenly made available exclusively to the second twin, who is then acutely transfused and suddenly becomes hypervolemic. In the presence of antepartum TTT, the 'stuck' donor twin is usually born second. Therefore, should intrapartum TTT supervene chronic prenatal TTT, it is this small donor twin (who may be expected to be anemic) who is paradoxically plethoric at birth (see Figure 3.10, pages 141–2).

Similar principles apply to the fetal death of one MC twin, whether from antepartum TTT or other causes (Figure 3.11, pages 142–3). Relationships between the surviving twin and total placental circulation are radically altered if superficial anastomoses are present, and acute hypovolemia and hypotension often affect the survivor.

It is likely that such events (for example, the rapidly changing blood pressures) may cause much of the parenchymal organ damage found in most surviving twins, although the older literature implicates intravascular transfer of thrombotic material in this process. However, the putative mechanism(s) by which thromboplastins are transferred from the dead twin to the survivor is far from clear, and the concept is disputed by some authorities who cogently note that dead twins are incapable of pumping anything out of their vascular systems.

Methods for selective termination of MC twins should take into account the potential presence of vascular anastomoses. The intracardiac injection of toxic chemicals in one twin may shortly be followed by the death of both fetuses if the agent reaches the other twin via these anastomoses. Moreover, the sudden death of the terminated twin may cause acute hemodynamic changes in the intended survivor if the circulations are connected.

At present, it is recommended that selective termination of MC twins use methods that achieve complete segregation of the two circulations to minimize the complications resulting from vascular connections. This may best be accomplished by selective delivery of the designated abnormal fetus by hysterotomy, cord ligation or placement of thrombogenic coils in the cord vessels of the abnormal twin. Regardless, all therapies for TTT are considered experimental at present.

Mechanisms of acardius

Acardiac twins are rare in MC pregnancies. By definition, the twin pair comprises a normal twin who acts as the 'pump' and an acardiac co-twin who is passively perfused by the 'pump' co-twin (Figures 3.12–3.15, pages 144–8). Acardiac fetuses occur relatively frequently in triplet pregnancies that may be MZ or DZ. Figure 3.12 a & b (page 144) illustrates the extremes of this condition: the former is more typical whereas the latter shows a more organized, but hydropic, acardiac fetus, probably representing an early phase of 'regression'.

At least two types of events may lead to the development of the acardiac state:

(1) The acardiac twin may be malformed *ab initio*. In support of this concept is the fact that up to 50% of acardiac twins are chromosomally abnormal whereas their corresponding pump twins are chromosomally normal (an example of heterokaryotypia; see Part I, Section 1, *Some reasons why monozygotic twins are not identical*). As a component of the chromosomal abnormality, the acardiac twin may have a variety of problems (including congenital heart disease (Figure 3.12 c, page 144), other thoracic malformations and / or hydrops), any one of which would prove lethal to a singleton fetus. If vascular anastomoses are present, the malformed fetus may survive passively via reversed arterial perfusion from the pump twin. If no appropriate fetal vascular anastomoses are present, this sequence could well lead to fetus papyraceus or vanishing MC twins, depending upon how early in development the abnormal perfusion begins; or

(2) The stronger twin may 'overwhelm' the circulation of an anatomically normal but 'weaker' twin via vascular anastomoses, and succeed in reversing the direction of flow in the umbilical vessels of the smaller twin. This would represent a severe form of antepartum TTT. The presence of large a→a and v→v anastomoses without a→v anastomoses, which is the pattern that is always present in acardiac MC gestations, argues against an overwhelming TTT event.

Acardiac twins have been diagnosed early in gestation, but the initiating events have never been witnessed. The explanations presented above are as yet unproven although, in some form, both mechanisms probably occur. The extent of visceral abnormality in the acardiac twin does not remain static, but may become more severe as the fetus continues to be passively perfused. When reversed perfusion is present, organs which have undergone early development may regress (Figure 3.13, page 145).

In the normal fetal circulation, the umbilical arteries carry deoxygenated denourished blood, predominantly from the brain, via veins of the fetal head and neck back to the placenta. There is little blood flow in the aortic isthmus between the left subclavian artery and ductus arteriosus. Therefore, any blood entering the descending thoracic aorta is largely transductal, having arrived in the right ventricle from the brain via preferential cross-flow in the right atrium (Figure 3.14 a, page 146).

Given this situation, it follows that the blood going to the acardiac twin via the unidirectional a→a anastomosis was originally destined for reoxygenation in the placental parenchyma, having already perfused the brain and heart of the pump twin. Likewise, venous blood leaves the acardiac twin via its umbilical vein and the v→v anastomosis.

This doubly perfused 'stale' blood is now preferentially routed to the brain of the pump twin before passing to its descending aorta and umbilical arteries. On reaching the chorionic plate, it may either perfuse the placental parenchyma or pass yet again to the acardiac twin. In theory, a proportion of the entire circulating volume of the twins could repeatedly perfuse the bodies of both before being replenished by one passage through the villous tree. Such an occurrence may well have a deleterious effect on brain development in the pump twin (see Figure 3.14 a, page 146).

In some respects, the a→v anastomosis of antepartum TTT is physiologically sound. However, the reversed a→a flow in the acardiac twin is basically unphysiological. As Ballantyne has so aptly noted, the acardiac twin "...will become a pensioner upon his brother's bounty." In effect, "... one of the organisms is a maternal parasite, while the other is a parasite upon this parasite." In such a vascular arrangement, the metabolic needs of the entire acadiac fetus are not adequately met, and a regressive type of fetal development supervenes. Moreover, the twice-circulated blood is not likely to have a beneficial effect on the growth and development of the pump twin.

The most severe defect in the acardiac fetus is usually seen at the cranial pole. This region has high metabolic requirements for oxygen and is farthest from the iliac region, the point of entry of blood into the arterial tree. In some acardiac cases, the placental arterial connection appears vitelline in type. Similar principles are then applicable, but the result may be acardiac fetuses with relatively greater representation of the cranial pole.

The acardiac twin most commonly consists of a torso and regressed legs (see Figures 3.12 a and 3.13, pages 144–5). Blood leaves the acardiac fetus by reversed flow in the umbilical vein and returns to the pump twin via a superficial $v \rightarrow v$ anastomosis. It is not clear how much of the placenta near the acardiac twin is perfused by its pump co-twin. The venous blood returning from the acardiac twin to the pump twin admixes with the remainder of the returning placental venous blood (see Figure 3.14, pages 146–7). Thrombosis is sometimes seen in the anastomotic vessels, which may indicate a risk for organ infarction in the pump twin.

The burden of perfusing the acardiac twin often causes cardiac failure in the pump twin together with the onset of hydrops; the mortality rate is high. Methods have been proposed to alleviate the cardiac decompensation by antepartum occlusion of the cord of the acardiac twin (Figure 3.15, page 148). These methods, however, are still under investigation. As with other types of fetal surgery, achieving adequate tocolysis remains a problem.

Monochorionic placental vascular patterns and perinatal outcomes

Growth discordance, TTT and TRAP are among several complications of MC twins that can be ascribed to particular placental vascular anastomotic patterns. In a retrospective clinicopathological study of 69 MC twin pregnancies, vascular anatomy was linked to several selected perinatal outcome parameters (Figure 3.16, pages 149–51). Growth discordance was reported to be due to unequal venous sharing. True antepartum TTT was found in twins whose placentas contained $a \rightarrow v$ anastomoses, often in the absence of compensatory $a \leftrightarrow a$ or $v \leftrightarrow v$ anastomoses. A great majority of perinatal morbidity and mortality occurred in this group (see Figure 3.16).

As there are several possible mechanisms whereby MC twins may show significant growth discordance, it is difficult to give parents sound advice as to the chances of growth catch-up on the basis of scientific data. This is because there have been few large-scale longitudinal studies of postnatal growth in twins of known zygosity, chorionicity and placental vascular status. A single case of growth follow-up is shown in Figure 3.17 (pages 151–2). Available data from the Louisville Twin Study, and a field study conducted at the Twins Day Festival in Twinsburg, Ohio, indicate that catch-up growth does indeed occur by adolescence. However, many factors influence the rate of catch-up growth, and these are presumably related to the various causes of the initial discordance.

Discordance for congenital anomalies in monozygotic twins

As already described (see Part I, Section 1, *Some reasons why monozygotic twins are not identical*), postzygotic events may cause MZ twin pairs to be discordant for chromosomal abnormalities, patterns of X-chromosome inactivation and gene imprinting.

Acardiac twins arise, directly or indirectly, because of the presence of vascular anastomoses in MC placentas. Conjoined twins are unique to MC, MZ twins (see *Monochorionic monoamniotic twins*).

Apart from these special mechanisms, many pairs of MZ twins are discordant for a variety of malformations that also occur in singletons and DZ twins, and which do not have a simple or straightforward genetic basis, but are most probably multifactorial in origin. These malformations include neural tube defects (see Figure 1.10), omphalocele (Figure 3.18, page 153), symmelia, holoprosencephaly (Figure 3.19 a, page 153), cleft lip and palate (Figure 3.19 b, page 153), and amniotic band syndrome. It is not clear how these discordant events arise, but the apparently unaffected co-twin on occasions has a much less severe manifestation of the same disease. This implies that the predisposition to malformation may be present in the whole zygote, but is differentially expressed in each of the twins. Congenital heart disease is a special consideration as some types of this disease may be caused by abnormal flow patterns during embryogenesis, and MC twins are particularly prone to such abnormal patterns.

At present, it has not been ascertained whether differential expression of a disease or condition is a stimulus to the twinning process. A clearer picture of the mechanisms underlying discordance in twins in terms of severity of expression of a given anomaly may lead to a new and better understanding of the initiating events that precede splitting of the inner cell mass. Equally, it may allow identification of relationships between anomalies that were previously not thought to be related. In the pair of MZ twins shown in Figure 1.10, for example, one twin has anencephaly whereas her co-twin has multiple thoracic hemivertebrae as the sole anomaly. Such discordance suggests that these two disorders probably have the same underlying causes, but differing expres-

sions presumably depending on the degree of abnormal development of the notochord.

Additional study of other discordant MZ twin pairs should provide further useful insights into the wider spectra of other well-known congenital malformations and syndromes.

From the practical point of view, THE ANTEPARTUM ULTRASOUND DIAGNOSIS OF TWINS DISCORDANT FOR MAJOR MALFORMATION DOES NOT NECESSARILY INDICATE THAT THEY ARE DZ AND THEREFORE DC. If selective termination is contemplated, there are risks to the intended survivor if placentation is MC (see Part I, Section 1, *Reproductive technology and multiple births*).

Management of complications of monochorionic twin pregnancy

In general, effective management of MC pregnancies depends on appreciation of the probably close vascular interdependence of the MC twin pairs. Hence, the interventional methods used in cases of DC twins and singletons may not be appropriate for MC twins. Indeed, the aim of intervention in the latter is to improve perfusion in both fetuses or to isolate the two circulations.

The principal problems in the management of MC pregnancy are recognition of the different causes of growth discordance, diagnosis of antepartum TTT and TRAP if present, and selective termination of one fetus in circumstances of severe fetal anomaly or impending fetal death to forestall organ infarction of the survivor. MC, MA twins are prone to further special risks (see below). These issues are even more complex in cases of triplets and HOMPs, where affected twin fetuses may be MZ and MC in relation to normal fetuses.

Pathology in monoamniotic twin pregnancy

In addition to the placental vascular risks of mono-chorionicity in both MC,DA and MC,MA twins mentioned above, MA twins are also at risk of cord complications. As both twins exist within one amniotic sac, their cords may become entangled and twisted to the extent that one or both fetal circulations are impaired (Figure 3.20, page 154; see also Figures 2.9–2.11). The condition is not always fatal, although both fetuses may die of asphyxia if complex cord braids or knots are formed. Alternatively, winding of the cord of one twin around the body of the other may result in a single fetal death.

It is axiomatic that a prolapsed or nuchal cord associated with the first-born MA twin may, in fact, belong to the second twin who is, during the interval prior to delivery, at risk of asphyxia and / or exsanguination if that cord is occluded, clamped or cut. This is especially true when MA twins occur as components of triplets or other HOMPs.

An interesting and unusual phenomenon in MA twin pairs is the protection of one twin from the effects of fetal oliguria / anuria when the other twin has normal urine production. In singleton fetuses, oliguria may be caused by bilateral renal agenesis / dysgenesis, urinary tract obstruction or infantile polycystic kidney disease. The result is 'mechanical' deformation, the so-called Potter, or oligohydramnios, syndrome, the lethal feature of which is pulmonary hypoplasia. The mechanical effects are caused by absent or severely reduced amniotic fluid volumes. In twins and HOMPs, similar findings are seen when the affected fetus lies in a separate sac, in particular, a DC sac. However, in the case of MA twins, both share a single amniotic sac, the volume of which can be adequately maintained by the urine production of only one twin.

In such an instance, the abnormal co-twin may produce no urine, yet show none of the mechanical deformations of oligohydramnios. The diagnosis of bilateral renal agenesis / dysgenesis, urinary tract obstruction or infantile polycystic kidney disease is therefore difficult to establish in a neonate who does not have oligohydramnios syndrome, but presents only with oliguria / anuria.

Conjoined twinning

This is the result of late and incomplete twin formation at the latest possible moment when the embryonic axis is being laid down (see Figure 1.3). The theoretical embryogenetic mechanisms of conjoined twinning and some examples are shown in Figures 3.21 and 3.22 (pages 155–62). Although the precise timing of conjoined twins is unknown, teratogenic animal experiments indicate that the 'decision' for such a formation is made shortly before the event takes place. Therefore, it is presumed that the zygote rapidly reorganizes into two closely apposed body axes and, subsequently, proceeds to develop two body plans, either complete or incomplete, within one ectodermal covering. Conjoined twins are usually MA, and around 75% are female. A surprising number occur in triplet pregnancies.

Newer anatomical classifications for conjoined twinning have recently been proposed, based on the likely three-dimensional relationships between the two fetal body plans during early embryogenesis. Previous classifications have been solely descriptive, based on the anatomical zones of coalescence and without consideration of the early embryological events of axiation and gastrulation. Knowledge of zones of contiguity is important in the decision-making process for potential surgical separation. Conjoined twins also yield important information on the mechanisms of normal and abnormal embryogenesis. What follows is an explanation of the anatomical types of conjoined twinning according to their embryogenesis. Readers are referred to standard texts for full documentation of the classical types of conjoined twins.

In general, the body axes of conjoined twins are arranged in one of two patterns:

(1) More or less side by side, as in dicephalus and diprosopus; or

(2) Orientations with the notochordal axes separated as far apart as possible, as in all other forms of conjoined twins.

Presumably, formation of the notochordal axes and the events of gastrulation are strongly defined by developmental genes, and these processes are so fundamental to early embryogenesis that they need to proceed as undisturbed and independently as possible, judging by the physical restrictions within the anatomical confines of conjoined twins.

However, in most instances of conjoined twins, complete independence of the two body axes is not possible. Furthermore, the two axes emit mutually interfering inductive developmental signals, which are both confusing to and difficult to interpret by the major organs of the simultaneously developing body zones. Of great importance in understanding the ultimate anatomical arrangements that result is the fact that the two closely apposed embryos may interfere with the normal processes of flexion, and headfold and tailfold formation.

Three main types of abnormal internal organ formation are produced by the disturbed anatomical and embryological relationships described above:

(1) Major overlap of organ fields, with coalescence of the liver, heart, intestinal tract and skeleton, as seen in thoracopagus;

(2) Failure of organ formation ('interaction aplasia'), including neural tube defect and omphalocele, as seen in dicephalus and diprosopus conjoined twins; and

(3) Formation of 'new' coalesced axes, as seen in the faces of janiceps and pelvic girdles of ischiopagus conjoined twins.

A minority of conjoined twins have minimal zones of coalescence and can be surgically separated. In the remainder, separation can only be achieved, often in stages, with the unequal allocation of organs and zones between the two separated twins. In some cases, one twin appears undergrown or malformed compared with the other, and management is aimed at saving the more completely formed twin. Regardless, the outcomes are not always predictable (see Part III, *Conjoined twinning*).

The surgical separation of conjoined twins is complex, and associated with major ethical and technical difficulties. In recent years, antepartum ultrasound diagnosis has led to more frequent early diagnosis of the lethal forms of conjoined twinning, with the use of pregnancy termination in many cases, and detailed plans for the delivery and postnatal management of potentially separable pairs.

Higher-order multiple pregnancy (HOMP)

This condition is relatively rare among naturally conceived pregnancies; the first review of triplet pregnancies was published as late as 1988. There is currently a growing international concern regarding the rising numbers of HOMPs that result from various forms of ART used to treat infertile couples. It is generally assumed that MZ twins, triplets and other multiples are rare in ART-induced pregnancies, but this is not the case. Contrary to expectations, MZ twins are found in 10–12% of all ART pregnancies, many of which are subject to the complications of MC placentation. In spontaneously conceived HOMPs, the rate of MZ and MC twinning is also high, with an excess of female MZ twins. Few detailed series have been reported in the literature.

HOMPs are at an exceptionally high risk of preterm delivery and its complications, leading to astronomical costs in neonatal care. In many centers, HOMPs resulting from ART are offered selective reduction down to triplets or twins, thereby lowering, but not eliminating, the rates of preterm delivery and even of growth restriction in the remaining fetuses.

Accurate antepartum determination of chorionicity is important in HOMPs (see Figures 2.1–2.3 and 2.15) as all of the complications of MC placentation may and do occur. In most cases, only the twin pair among three, four or more fetuses is involved in TTT, TRAP or MC, MA placentation, although complications such as hydramnios, fetal death and preterm delivery may adversely affect the remaining fetus(es). Unfortunately, delineation of the anatomically specific boundaries of each fetus and its sac is much more difficult and complex in such cases than in twin pregnancies. Interventional therapy requires much skill in ultrasonography as well as in fetal surgery.

In Table 3.3, the details of placentation and zygosity for 46 sets of spontaneously conceived triplets indicate that significant numbers are MZ (including MC) twins with an excess of females, and high mortality rates due to TTT and preterm delivery. Spontaneously conceived quadruplets and quintuplets are rare, and their zygosity and chorionicity only rarely reported. The placentas of HOMPs are discussed in Part II, Section 1, *Examination of HOMP placentas,* and illustrated in Part IV.

Table 3.3 Chorionicity and zygosity of 46 sets of spontaneously conceived triplets

Zygosity	MZ		DZ		TZ	
Placentation	*n*	*%*	*n*	*%*	*n*	*%*
MC	7	58	0	—	0	—
DC	4	33	17	71	0	—
TC	1	8	7	29	10	100
Total	12	100	24	100	10	100
Placentation	MC		DC		TC	
Zygosity	*n*	*%*	*n*	*%*	*n*	*%*
MZ	7	100	4	19	1	6
DZ	0	—	17	81	7	39
TZ	0	—	0	—	10	56
Total	7	100	21	100	18	100

Data are derived from Machin GA, Bamforth F. Zygosity and placental anatomy in 15 consecutive sets of spontaneously conceived triplets. *Am J Med Genet* 1996;61:247–52 and C. Derom, personal communication

Part 11 PRACTICAL ASPECTS

Section 1 How to examine twin and higher-order multiple pregnancy placentas

Introduction

There are two fundamental objectives in examining the placentas of multiple pregnancies:

(1) To correlate the clinical obstetric features with the anatomy and pathology of the placenta(s), in particular, with respect to chorionicity and the presence of specific vascular anastomotic patterns in MC placentas; and

(2) To determine zygosity where possible.

Both of these objectives may have legal implications.

Placentas are preferably examined in the fresh state rather than after formalin fixation. Fresh placentas can best be sampled for microbiology and DNA zygosity studies, and vascular perfusion studies are more successful when the placentas are fresh. Cords should be identified by birth order, using ties or cord clamps. The least equivocal system entails placing one marker on the cord of twin A, two on that of B, and so on.

As a minimum, clinical information on the dated pathology requisition slip should include obstetric complications, mode of delivery, gender and birth weights as well as the date of the last menstrual period and best obstetric estimate of gestational age based on early ultrasound. A logical stepwise examination proceeds as follows.

Naked-eye diagnosis of chorionicity

If the placental disks and membranes are separate, they almost invariably represent DC twinning. Although the great majority of MC placentas consist of a single disk, on occasions, cases have been described with two disks or with a bipartite disk with a minimal amount of bridging tissue (see Figure 3.5).

In the case of a single placental mass, this may be a fused DC or truly MC placenta. To distinguish these two forms of placentation, the membranous septum is carefully examined with the naked eye, after which the septal components in one limited area are gently pulled apart into their constituent layers. This leaves the other areas intact for later histological sampling. In some cases, the septum will have been severely disrupted during delivery, for example, by cord avulsion.

The fused DC septum consists of two layers of chorion and two of amnion. The individual chorion layers often cannot be separated. The membranous chorion is firmly continuous with the chorionic plate of the placenta proper, from which it cannot be detached. (This area corresponds to the delta sign that is often clearly seen on early obstetric ultrasonography.)

In contrast, in MC,DA placentas, the septum consists of only two amniotic layers, with no chorionic components, and is thin and fragile. Moreover, whereas the *DC septum is translucent* (Figure 4.1a, page 163), the *MC,DA septum is transparent* (Figure 4.1b, page 163). Simple comparison of the structure (Figure 4.1c & d, page 163) is within the capability of all healthcare professionals, and there is no reason why this distinction cannot be made in the delivery room. For such a procedure, the services of a perinatal pathologist are not required.

Many obstetric units routinely submit all twin placentas for full investigation, and the present authors endorse such a practice. If chorionic status is not adequately documented in the delivery room and / or laboratory, the opportunity to record MC status at birth (indicating monozygosity) will be missed; this information may prove invaluable later in the lives of the twins (see Part III).

To summarize, the fused DC septum is thick and translucent, comprises four layers and is firmly attached to the placenta. In contrast, the MC, DA septum is thin, transparent and friable, and comprises only the two amniotic layers; its base is not firmly attached to the placenta and is more likely to be disrupted to some degree during delivery.

The absence of a strongly attached chorionic component is usually clearly evident, but distinguishing between MC, DA and MC, MA placentation may be difficult when the membranes are disrupted. The distinction between DC and MC placentation can usually be made by naked-eye examination (see Figure 4.1), and should always be confirmed by microscopy.

MC, MA placentation is occasionally overdiagnosed. If the septum of an MC, DA placenta has been disrupted, the amniotic remnants are usually gathered around the insertion points of both cords. By laying these remnants back into their most likely correct anatomical positions, it can then usually be appreciated that there is too much amniotic membrane between the cord insertions for the placentation to have been MC, MA. Indeed, it may be possible to find some zones where the two amniotic layers are still apposed, and these areas should be sampled with membrane rolls (see histology section below).

If one or both cords have been avulsed and taken the amnion with them, it may be impossible to distinguish between MC, DA and MC, MA placentation. *However, in truly MC, MA placentas, the amnion lies flat on the chorionic plate between the cord insertions and is less likely to be disrupted than an MC, DA septum.* Intertwined cords are found in approximately half of all MC, MA placentas.

Weights and measures

Placentas are then weighed and measured. General features are noted, such as the exact sites of cord insertions, or the presence of chorioamnionitis, infarction or hemorrhage. Clinicopathological correlations may be sought with fetal disorders such as growth discordance, malformation, hydrops and fetal death.

Histology of chorionicity

Histological confirmation of dichorionicity is now performed. With DC placentas, standard blocks may be taken for general histological assessment of any pathological areas noted on gross examination. With MC placentas, no histological blocks are taken until vascular studies are completed (see below).

In the case of fused DC placentas, T-junction septal samples must be taken (Figure 4.2, page 164). However, because of the fragility of MC, DA placentas (Figure 4.3 a, page 165), T-junction samples are not easily obtainable and should, in any case, not be attempted until injection studies have been completed. Equally acceptable and much simpler is the preparation of membrane rolls from the fresh septum (Figure 4.3 b–e, pages 165–6). *It is mandatory to document MC status by microscopy as this will produce permanent evidence of monozygosity.*

Vascular injection of MC placentas

The vessels of MC placentas are now examined. Dye injection demonstrates the number and type of vascular anastomoses, and allows assessment of the ratio of venous sharing between the twins (Figure 4.4, pages 166–7; see also Figures 3.3–3.7 for the results of such studies).

Arterial and venous catheters are optimally inserted within 2–3 cm of the cord insertion. If there is cord avulsion or trauma to vessels in the chorionic plate, injection may still be possible into selected vessels on the chorionic plate itself. Catheters and syringes are primed with dye to minimize the presence of air bubbles.

Gentle transverse cuts through the cord stroma allow exposure and partial transection of selected vessels, which can then be dilated with a probe to facilitate passage of the catheters. If the vessels are contorted, the gentle use of a probe may act as an introducer by straightening the bends to facilitate insertion of the catheter. It may be necessary to massage blood and clots from the chorionic surface vessels (particularly the veins) through the transected umbilical vessel(s) before catheterization.

The likely pathophysiological events determine which vessels are to be catheterized. For instance, in a case of suspected TTT, it is sensible to catheterize an artery of the donor and a vein of the recipient, thereby highlighting areas of potential a → v anastomosis. It is useful to remember that, when the artery meets the vein on the surface, they meet 'nose-to-nose,' and the artery is 'naked' or unaccompanied by a vein. The same is true for the veins which anastomose deep in the cotyledon with the artery. In the presence of growth discordance, the veins of both twins should be injected to appreciate the difference in the sizes of the fields of perfusion.

Catheters are tied in position to prevent leakage. *The findings of injection studies should be recorded by color photography.* The paths of flow of the colored dye particles can also be traced on microscopy (Figure 4.4 e, page 167). Finally, there is little point in performing injection studies unless the cords of the twins have been identified.

Routine histology of MC placentas

Routine histological sections are taken from MC placentas. Patterns of dye distribution in various perfusion zones can be confirmed by the presence of dye particles in villous vessels (see Figure 4.4 e).

Tissue sampling for zygosity testing

Tissue samples may be taken for DNA extraction and zygosity testing. Strictly speaking, this is required only in like-sexed DC twins (who may be either DZ or MZ). However, as there is sufficient research interest in the events surrounding the causation of MZ twins, it is prudent to collect DNA samples from MC twin placentas as well.

A 1-ml (cc) cube of chorionic placenta is sufficient. A chorion sample is best taken close to the point of cord insertion and near to the fetal surface to minimize maternal decidual contamination. Umbilical cord and amnion can also be used for DNA extraction. (For details of zygosity-testing methods, see Part II, Section 2.) There is little point in performing zygosity testing in HOMPs unless the cords of the fetuses have been identified.

Examination of higher-order multiple pregnancy placentas

This procedure is an extension of the methods just described, but is more complex. Cord identification is vital for success. Combinations of MZ, DZ, MC and DC placental relationships are seen; the objectives remain the determination of zygosity and delineation of clinicopathological events. (Figures 4.5–4.9, pages 168–74, show examples of typical cases.)

Selective-reduction multiple pregnancies

In the event of HOMPs resulting from *in vitro* fertilization (infrequent) or ovulation induction (much more common), selective reduction(s) in the second trimester results in papyraceous fetuses that can usually be identified around the edges of the placental disks of the surviving fetuses (Figure 4.10, page 175).

Summary

The methods described here are relatively simple, inexpensive and not excessively time-consuming.

Eventually, this type of examination could be carried out by trained pathology assistants. The results will add immeasurably to the understanding of events occurring in all twin pregnancies, particularly MC pregnancies. A routine mechanistic anatomical pathological study alone may not always provide the quality of information that may otherwise be gathered by the use of several simple techniques in the problem-based knowledge-generating protocol outlined here.

Section 2 How to test twins for zygosity
Fiona Bamforth

Introduction

It is surprising how unusual it is for twins and / or their parents to either know their zygosity or understand its implications. Unlike-sexed twins are usually DZ (but see Part I, *Some reasons why mono-zygotic twins are not identical*), and all MC twins are MZ. However, around one-quarter of DC twins are MZ.

The main sources of difficulty are:

(1) The widespread belief, even among trained obstetricians, that all DC twins are DZ;

(2) That chorionicity is not always noted at birth and parents are not informed that MC twins are always MZ; and

(3) That many parents think that their twins must be 'identical' in every way before they can be considered to be MZ.

Why twins should know their zygosity is discussed in Part III.

A brief review of methods for zygosity testing

Except in the rare events of postzygotic hetero-karyotypia, differential imprinting, point mutation or highly skewed X-chromosome inactivation, MZ pairs have all of their genes in common. In contrast, DZ twins (if homopaternal) share, on average, only half the alleles for which their parents are hetero-zygous.

All methods of zygosity testing seek to show allelic discordance, thus proving dizygosity. Failure to demonstrate dizygosity at many alleles allows the diagnosis of monozygosity by exclusion, the degree of statistical certainty depending on the number of loci tested and allele frequencies at those loci. Even when the polypeptide products of multiple gene loci (for example, blood-group antigens, red cell enzymes, and plasma proteins and enzymes) are tested, the statistical certainty may not be high.

Gene analysis can be performed directly at the level of DNA, testing as many loci as necessary to reach the diagnosis. DNA methods use segments of DNA that show highly variable lengths or sequences that are inherited co-dominantly. They may be detectable as restriction fragment length polymorphisms (RFLPs) or as variable number tandem repeat sequences (VNTRs). These inherited patterns may be tested one locus at a time (as in blood- and serum-marker tests) or by simultaneous locus analysis (Figure 5.1, page 176).

If a single-locus probe is used and the parents between them have four different alleles at a given locus, there is only a 1:4 chance that DZ twins will inherit the same allelic pattern (Figure 5.2, page 176). If two single-locus probes are used, then the likelihood of concordance is $^1/_4 \times {}^1/_4$, or $^1/_{16}$. With three or four probes, the likelihood is $^1/_{64}$ or $^1/_{256}$, respectively. Even when the parents have four different alleles for each probe, many probes have to be used to obtain statistical certainty. In other cases, analysis may be less informative because the number of alleles at a given locus in the parents is less than four, thus reducing the discriminatory power of the test.

Multilocus probes are used to detect VNTRs that are present at many loci throughout the genome. Because they are highly variable and numerous, VNTRs are one of the best methods for zygosity testing. Siblings (including DZ twins) share around 70% of their alleles when tested with a multilocus probe. In the experience of the present author, it is sufficient to use two multilocus VNTR probes at low stringency. If doubt arises, a third VNTR probe may be used at either high or low stringency.

Sample procurement and processing

DNA can be extracted from any type of nucleated cell. Cord blood or placental tissue can be used after birth, and chorionic villus samples, amniocytes or cord blood samples can be used for prenatal diagnosis. Indeed, the survival of DNA in macerated stillborn fetuses is sufficiently good that analysis may even be achieved after fetal death (including fetus papyraceus). There may be enough DNA in mouthwash or cheek mucosal brush samples for use in polymerase chain reaction (PCR)-based methods, which are usually single-locus probes.

Specimens can be taken for zygosity testing at the time of placental examination. The fetal surface should be used to avoid contamination by maternal decidua (Figure 5.3, page 177). As formalin fixation tends to degrade DNA, fresh tissue is preferable. Adequate DNA is often extractable from paraffin-processed tissue blocks.

When using fixed tissue, DNA extraction should be carried out gently, avoiding vigorous shaking, vortexing or homogenization. After extraction, DNA can be stored for long periods at $4\,°C$, $-20\,°C$ or $-70\,°C$. Peripheral blood samples are also convenient for zygosity testing. Whole blood anticoagulated with ethylenediaminetetraacetic acid (EDTA) may be sent by courier to the testing laboratory to arrive within 3–4 days testing. Samples should not be frozen or excessively heated.

Recommended method for zygosity testing

With the standard Southern blot technique, we routinely use VNTR probes 3'HVR and YNH24 (Figure 5.4, pages 177–8) whereas INS310 and HMF-1 are used for additional testing, as necessary. More than one multilocus probe should be used because, by chance, a twin pair may appear to be MZ by one probe, but prove to be unequivocally DZ from the results of a second probe (Figure 5.5, page 179).

Probes 3'HVR and YNH24 may be used as single-locus probes at high stringency and as multilocus probes at low stringency. They are easy to use and may give results even when DNA quality is poor.

Potential technical problems include:

(1) Partial digestion, resulting in extra bands that vary within an MZ twin pair (Figure 5.6, page 179);

(2) Very poor DNA quality. In such an event, it is better to request a further sample;

(3) DNA concentrations should be roughly equal for each pair;

(4) Degraded DNA has a different electrophoretic mobility than intact DNA, leading to apparent mismatching (Figure 5.7, page 180); and

(5) By chance, some DZ twin pairs may have many alleles in common (see Figure 5.5).

In addition, MZ twins may be genetically discordant. **Thus, the gold standard for monozygosity is monochorionicity; the problems associated with DNA-based diagnosis can usually be resolved.** Zygosity testing is particularly useful in DZ pairs who, by chance, are phenotypically very similar (Figure 5.8, page 181).

Section 3 How to photograph twin faces for medical purposes
David Teplica

Introduction

Photographic images are useful in the assessment of twin zygosity and symmetry. Standardized techniques are required to produce photographs for scientific analysis. Home photographs may be misleading because of variability in lighting, positioning of the subject, film stock and camera equipment. To obviate such problems, the following guidelines have been distilled from the large body of photographic and technical literature. These methods will allow clinicians, parents and others to capture standardized facial images that are useful for scientific comparison.

The techniques described here were developed by the author and used to produce the Twinsburg Archive, the largest known repository of facial images of twins. Subjects between 4 and 94 years of age can be effectively studied. Younger children may not be able to concentrate sufficiently. Moreover, facial features are not fully expressed at an earlier age.

Several general principles apply:

(1) Subjects should be photographed separately;

(2) Subjects should be free of facial expressions such as smiling, grimacing or frowning;

(3) Photographs should be logged, dated and labelled to avoid confusion as to which images apply to which twin;

(4) Detailed consents should be obtained for rights to research or publication; and

(5) Subjects with dark skin pigmentation will require up to one *f*-stop of additional exposure.

Specific guidelines

Four categories of variables should be controlled:

Photographic environment

Subjects should be recorded without visible background objects. An unlit black background such as a flat black painted wall, dull black paper or flat black fabric may be used. Subjects should be comfortably seated in an erect posture. Stools or dental chairs are useful. Ambient light should be minimal to avoid variation in lighting balance, color or presence of shadows. Subjects' clothing should be draped out of view, using an 18% gray cloth to eliminate alterations of facial skin tones caused by light reflected from clothing.

Photographic equipment

A good-quality camera, lens and flash unit are optimal because of their durability. An adjustable tripod allows the lens to be positioned horizontal to the eyes of the subjects. Ideally, three undiffused strobe-flash lights are positioned to give even facial illumination. None are mounted on the camera. Two flash units are placed at 45° from the line between the camera and the subject's head. The third, less important, flash unit is positioned above and behind the head to provide 'rim light' to separate the subjects from the background. Incandescent bulbs with blue filters can be substituted if necessary.

A camera-mounted flash may be used, with the angle of light coming from above the lens. The same camera body and lens should be used over time to avoid the perceptual changes that result when varied equipment is used. A standard 105-mm lens is optimal. Lenses with higher angles of capture can introduce facial distortion.

Shutter speed should be set to the standard 'synch flash' speed and locked in this position to avoid error. The *f*-stop is determined by film speed. Longer shutter times and larger apertures decrease the amount of detail captured. The highest possible value (smallest aperture) will ensure that the maximum amount of anatomical detail is in focus.

Preparation and positioning of subjects

All make-up and jewellery should be removed. Hair should be fastened so as not to obscure facial detail. Standardized views of the facial anatomy are taken to avoid head tilt. The Frankfort horizontal plane is determined by palpation of the superior aspects of both external auditory meatuses and the most inferior points on the inferior orbital rims. The photographer then orients the subject's face so that the Frankfort plane is parallel to the floor. After this, the subject is asked to remain still. The correct position can be checked prior to each shot.

A constant distance should be maintained between the optical center of the lens and a line connecting the two inferior orbital rims. The face is best recorded at reproduction ratios of 1:8 to 1:10. Using a Nikon 105-mm lens, for example, the lens should be approximately 110 cm (43 inches) from the infraorbital rim.

Six anatomical images should be obtained from each subject (Figure 6.1, pages 182–3): frontal, with the subject looking straight at the lens; right and left obliques, with the subject rotated 45° from the frontal, but continuing to look straight ahead; right and left profiles, with the subject rotated 90° from the frontal, but looking straight ahead; and the 'worm's-eye view', which is a frontal orientation with the head tipped up 45° from the Frankfort plane. If there are particular features such as nevi or anomalies, these can be recorded for each subject using specific views and close-ups as necessary.

Film and processing

Transparencies are better than prints because they are longer-lasting, can be used directly for presentations and are processed with a greater degree of color consistency. Scientific images are best captured on professional-grade film stock, which is rigidly controlled for variability by the manufacturers. Likewise, processing should be done by a fully professional, quality-controlled laboratory. Ektachrome® EPN 100 is one of the most accurate and consistent film stocks for human anatomical photography, although Kodachrome® emulsions appear to have the greatest longevity.

Examples

Photographs of the faces of MZ twin pairs are particularly useful in analyzing the processes of differentiation and migration of the complex embryonic components of the face. Genetic and environmental effects can be appreciated, as well as the plasticity involved and any evidence of mirroring phenomena. Close inspection shows unexpected degrees of similarity, which suggest that genetic influences on development, growth and aging are highly significant (Figures 6.2–6.4, pages 184–6).

Part III LIVES OF SOME TWINS
AND THEIR PARENTS

Introduction

It is difficult for a singleton to understand what it is like to be a twin; the opposite is also true. For most twins, whether they are MZ or DZ, life is individual and unique. In spite of this, twin pairs as well as the general population are prone to question whether two individuals are to be thought of as 'the twins' or as individual members of a twin pair. Without doubt, the answer is that they are both and therein lies the paradox. These same questions are also valid for triplets and other multiples.

On the basis of biology (and pathology), many aspects of 'twinness' generate fascinating and important questions. These include: How many twins develop their own language? Why do some apparently demonstrate mirror-imaging? Are some twins in some way psychically linked? Unfortunately, the exceedingly complex and variable nature of twinning and twin life make it impossible to provide accurate answers to these and other commonly asked questions.

In some cases, the inability to be specific as regards a given question is due to a lack of knowing the zygosity of the twin pair. Even when the issue is of great importance, few answers can be offered with certainty. We are as yet unable to provide parents with pair-specific prognostic advice regarding potential catch-up growth in twins with marked birth-weight discordance because many factors may relate to the discordance and these factors remain largely unknown if the placenta has not been examined in detail. Similarly, we are unable to state with certainty whether the twin who currently dominates the other will continue to do so, because the degree to which the temperaments of twins may vary within a pair, especially an MZ pair, is not fully understood.

Neither is it possible to predict with certainty the extent to which the two members of a twin pair will depend on each other, enhance or retard individuation, cooperate or compete, or like or hate each other. The list of unanswerable questions goes on and on. Innumerable patterns occur, and these patterns probably vary with the passage of time and changes of circumstances.

Parents' knowledge of twins

In addition to the many aspects concerning twins that remain unknown from the scientific point of view, there are scant data about parental knowledge of twins and the twinning process. During twin pregnancy and birth, it appears that the issue of zygosity does not arise and is not widely discussed. The main objective is to have a good pregnancy and an uncomplicated delivery of both twins. It is only in the newborn period that zygosity comes to the fore. The first questions that parents are usually asked tend to be about the twins' zygosity, but the parents usually have no answers. Indeed, 'zygosity' is often considered a 'foreign' word and parents commonly are questioned in terms of identicality. From this point onwards, parents want to know how to help their twins become individuals, but do not know how to do so. Will they dress their twins differently? How do they really feel about their twins?

Perhaps some clues may be gleaned from the naming of twins. For example, are the names given to twins different according to their presumed zygosity? In a study of a series of 211 twin pairs, 42 pairs (20%) were found to have names which began with the same letter:

Aaron & Adam, Alvina & Angela, Amanda & Alycia, Braydon & Bryce, Caleigh & Christina, Carla & Carrie, Carmen & Colin, Colby & Cooper, Daniel & Dustin, Darren & Darrell, Derek & Dylan, Garry & Glen, Jacqueline & Janice, Jacqueline & Jennifer, Jacqueline & Jennifer, Janelle & Julie, Jennifer & Joshua, Jeremy & Jordan, Jesse & Joel, Justin & Jenna, Karin & Kristin, Kathleen & Kevin, Kelsey &

Kylie, Kelsi & Kaysi, Laura & Leanne, Matthew & Michael, Melissa & Mark, Mitchell & Michael, Monique & Marc, Monique & Michelle, Nicole & Noel, Patrick & Phillip, Rachel & Rebecca, Raenell & Rhonda, Sharleen & Sandra, Stacey & Scott, Stephanie & Sarah, Stephanie & Susanna, Tara & Tanya, Teagan & Tierra, Todd & Travis and Zan & Zoe. Probably the most confusing pairing in this group was Ashley Lynne & Lesley Anne.

Among twins with matching names, there were girl–boy pairs who are clearly DZ. In no instance was there a discernible or logical pattern to the naming, such as might be expected if a given letter were used for girls and another for boys, or if like letters were used for MZ twins and unlike letters for DZ twins.

It is clear that zygosity need not be a factor in the early relationships that parents establish with their twins. It is not known whether or to what extent these patterns affect the behavior of the twins. There are no data for the manner in which twins regard their naming process, whether they quickly reject their given names once they go to school or adopt nicknames or, further, whether they take legal steps to change their given names to one more preferable to the individual. In spite of the lack of information on this and similar matters, the questions are valid. Clearly, more research is needed.

Nature and nurture in twins

Perhaps the area wherein questions most readily come to mind concerns twin similarity. As MZ twin pairs age, do they begin to look and behave more or less alike, or remain the same? Are all three processes possible? If so, how does gender affect the process? What about smoking and drinking? Do these activities affect aging and skin changes in twins at the same rate or to the same degree, and how do these changes differ from changes in

their non-twin siblings? If the genetic make-up of MZ twins is the same, does this fact determine the manner in which twins experience life, making or keeping them remarkably similar?

No definitive work has been published in this field. Even the collection of 6000 photographs contained in the Twinsburg archives, compiled by David Teplica with the collaboration of Donald and Louis Keith, fails to address these questions. Three sets of MZ twin pairs photographed over many years (Figure 7.1, pages 187–8) demonstrate that physical similarities remain exceptionally strong in these photographs, which were not taken with the intention of making comparisons. The figures referred to in Part II, Section 3, document the physical similarities of MZ twin pairs in detail.

As implied in Part I, *Some reasons why monozygotic twins are not identical*, questions of nature and nurture are not easy to answer. Several types of post-zygotic genetic and / or prenatal environmental (mostly placental) events can cause MZ twins to appear strikingly dissimilar at birth and prevent these dissimilarities from changing (see Figure 1.1).

Paradoxically, there is evidence that postnatal environmental events in MZ twins do not occur at random. Indeed, the postnatal environment and its events may be selected and experienced by behavioral traits that are partly or largely inherited. If this is so, then MZ twin pairs, including those reared apart, are likely to filter and select similar life experiences. MZ twins, for example, are likely to be concordant not only for whether they fought in the war in Vietnam, but also for whether they were wounded in action.

Furthermore, if genetic factors indeed control a variety of brain functions such as mood, behavior, perception and personality, then genetics may to some degree also determine the environmental experiences of MZ twins. If this is the case, MZ twin pairs may in fact become more alike with time, as they become molded by common selection and perception of experience. Admittedly, the evidence for this proposition is not extensive, but compelling examples of dramatic similarities between pairs of MZ twins reared apart have been gathered by Thomas Bouchard at the University of Minnesota.

Such is the power of twin studies in discriminating between the effects of genetic predisposition and environmental experience that a large multidisciplinary study is now contacting approximately 16 000 surviving male twin pairs who served in World War II. They will be questioned regarding concordance / discordance for a variety of important chronic diseases that affect the increasingly numerous elderly populations of developed countries, for example, Parkinson's disease, Alzheimer's disease, cancer and stroke.

Thus far, the issues of zygosity and chorionicity in this text have been presented from scientific and medical points of view. However, in this section, these same issues are looked at in terms of their consequences in the lives of MZ twins. Four groups of real-life stories have been taken from the files of one of the authors (GAM) to provide a more personal perspective of the subject.

Impact of zygosity on the lives of twins

Organ transplantation

MZ twins almost invariably have all their genes in common, including those determining histocompatibilty, a term which refers to one person's ability to detect tissue grafts received from another. Indeed, the ability to accept or reject a skin graft is an old-fashioned method of determining zygosity. In the event that one twin may require a graft or transplant of most types, an MZ co-twin is clearly the ideal donor candidate. On the basis of this

principle, some types of congenital defects, such as spina bifida and hypospadias, can be corrected in an affected newborn MZ twin by using skin grafts from the co-twin. In one case, extensive skin grafting of a spinal defect was possible with the use of donor skin from a stillborn MZ co-twin. In another case, circumcision of the normal twin provided enough skin to repair the hypospadias in his MZ co-twin.

In later life, kidney donation from MZ twins is an ideal means to avoid the complications of immuno-suppression administered to prevent transplant rejection. If for no other reason than the potential need for organ transplantation, all twins should know their zygosity. Above all, the misunderstandings that may arise from confusion over the precise meaning of 'identical' and of 'monozygotic' should be avoided, as clearly illustrated in the following case history.

A pair of male twins decided between themselves in early life that they were DZ because of:

(1) Opposite-handedness;

(2) Opposite hair whorls;

(3) Heterochromia iridis (differently colored irides of the eyes) in one twin whereas the co-twin had a normal iris color (Figure 7.2, page 189); and

(4) An extensive family history of twinning (which is usually associated with DZ twins).

When one twin lost all kidney function after eating toxic mushrooms, his co-twin gladly served as a live kidney transplant donor. The recipient was given full immunosuppression therapy for nearly 15 years simply because no one thought to question their zygosity. Later, both twins were full of consternation when DNA studies demonstrated that, despite their physical differences, they were in fact

MZ and the immunosuppression therapy had been completely unnecessary.

The issue of the twins' zygosity could and should have been fully investigated prior to transplant-ation. Fortunately, the recipient has subsequently been weaned from immunosuppression therapy, and now enjoys a considerable improvement in overall health with normal renal function.

Misassignment of zygosity at birth

The next two stories are further striking examples of misunderstandings as regards zygosity and placental structure.

After the birth of a pair of male twins (A and B), the parents were told that the twins must be DZ because they were DC. However, another male (C) was born in the same hospital that day, and the three newborn boys became inadvertently switched around in the nursery, such that A and C were taken home as a DZ twin pair, and B went home as a singleton. Twenty years later, C met B at school and remarked how closely B resembled his DZ twin A (Figure 7.3, page 190). Subsequent tests showed that A and B were in fact MZ twins, albeit DC (as are one-third of all MZ twins). The conse-quences for the three boys and their respective parents are virtually impossible to imagine.

On a happier note, one of the authors of this book (LGK) spent around 40 years wondering why he looked so much like his 'fraternal twin' (see Figure 7.1). Only when Professor Walter Nance obtained blood samples for zygosity analysis did the twins come to understand the practical implica-tions of being born with two placental disks (DC) and having 'identical' blood types. Their MZ status has been confirmed by full DNA analysis in paired laboratories of world renown.

Concordance of MZ twins for genetic diseases

MZ twins usually have the same genetic diseases. For example, MZ twins may both develop cancers that depend on a genetic predisposition, although the time of clinical expression may differ. In a typical scenario of such an occurrence, one twin with immunodeficiency (hyper-IgM hypogamma-globulinemia) developed extensive liver cancer at the age of 23 years (Figure 7.4a, page 190). His MZ twin was fully investigated, but showed no trace of cancer at that time. Within 1 year, however, the second twin developed the same type of wide-spread cancer (Figure 7.4b, page 190).

In this instance, the awareness of monozygosity did not prevent (or enhance) the development of clinical disease in the co-twin, although a know-ledge of the likelihood of a similar outcome was helpful. This is also true with the virtually simulta-neous development of certain types of childhood leukemias in MZ twins.

In the future, clinicians may be bold enough to carry out major surgery to excise potential areas of premalignancy in one MZ twin based on the strong presumption or proof that malignancy will eventually develop as it already has in the co-twin.

Impact of chorionicity on the lives of twins

Monochorionic twins have particularly high risks for morbidity and mortality for reasons already described in Part I, Section 3. To follow are three examples of such pregnancies and the manner in which precise data may lead to better results.

Twins who survived TTT, but exhibit developmental delay

Claudine and Jean-Pierre already had three children

when Claudine became pregnant again. At 17 weeks, twins were diagnosed by ultrasound. The technician thought they were probably MZ because only one placenta was present and the septal membrane was thin.

On recovering from their initial shock, the parents felt proud and excited. The other children thought that having twin siblings would be 'cool', and believed that the family was special because they were going to have twins. Everyone the couple knew was told the great news. They reorganized their home and bought a van. Claudine avidly read everything she could find concerning twins, wanting to do everything possible to have a successful pregnancy. She discussed the method of delivery with her obstetrician.

At 24 weeks, Claudine began to feel a worsening pain between her ribs and under her breasts. Her doctor believed that this was simply due to her small size (her height: 5 feet or 1.52 m) and the relatively large twin pregnancy. She asked for a second ultrasound examination, but her request was denied. Instead, she received a lecture on hospital budgets and abuse of tests.

Finally, however, because of persistent pain, an ultrasound examination was ordered for her stomach and gallbladder, but the technician refused to examine the twins because this had not been requested by the physician. She finally called the head of obstetrics at her local hospital, who scheduled an appointment.

The night before that appointment, Claudine's pain became so severe that she called the local emergency service and was asked by their staff to come in. Two fetal monitors showed that the twins were in distress, and she was given betamethasone. As Claudine was then in labor, she was transferred to a large city hospital which had a neonatal intensive care unit (NICU).

Ultrasonography at this time showed that twin A (Mathieu) had hydramnios and twin B (Michel) had oligohydramnios. Both demonstrated non-reactive non-stress tests (NSTs), and the doctors suspected TTT. An hour later, the twins were born by emergency Cesarean section under epidural anesthesia.

At birth, Mathieu weighed 1065 g and Michel weighed 950 g. Not only had Claudine and Jean-Pierre never seen such tiny premature infants, but they never imagined that they would have to assume a parenting role for such tiny children. Born without warning, would they survive? Would one or both of them die? How much would all of their care cost, both emotionally and financially?

Claudine visited the NICU for the first time the next day. The twins were receiving complex technological care for their respiratory distress, prematurity and the consequences of TTT. Claudine's first reaction was one of guilt that her physical pain had been transferred to the twins. There they lay, spreadeagled in their isolettes, blind-folded because of the bililights, attached to intravenous tubes, monitors and ventilators. She could neither pick them up nor cuddle them and she simply felt so SORRY.

As soon as the immediate neonatal complications of prematurity had been dealt with (including respiratory distress syndrome, bronchopulmonary dysplasia and retinopathy of prematurity in both twins, and intraventricular hemorrhage in Mathieu), it became apparent that both Mathieu, the recipient, and Michel, the donor, would have significant developmental delay. Indeed, Michel has cerebral palsy and spastic quadriplegia. The developmental pediatrician has had long meetings with the parents to explain the guarded prognosis for normal brain function. The news of the cerebral palsy was a severe blow to both parents; Claudine began to fall apart, but Jean-Pierre, being less involved in their day-to-day care, took the news rather better than did his wife. The future appeared to be bleak and the struggles endless.

However, both parents have regathered their strength and are now determined advocates for their twins. They have called on a multitude of support agencies, seeking all the information, equipment and personal support they can find to give their twins the maximum opportunity to develop their potential. All of this work has finally begun to pay off, as Michel is now making steady progress (Figure 7.5, page 191). Mathieu is an amusing young man who is happy and outgoing, and always trying to make the family laugh. Michel is more reserved, but always tries to imitate his twin. He is frustrated by his immobility, but receives great support.

The past 2 years have brought to this family a series of events that few others have experienced: the great expectations, the terrible crises, the episodes of despair and hope, the exhaustion and, finally, the steady determination to overcome. In the aftermath, Claudine admits that her one regret is that she did not seek out another doctor to ensure better prenatal care when she first experienced the pain, sensed that something was wrong, but received no support from her physicians.

Critique

Several points stand out in this story. After the shock of learning of the twin pregnancy, there was great enthusiasm and forward planning for the birth, but no attention was paid by the physicians to the potential for MC placentation indicated by the thin septal membrane. Although the parents had read a number of books on the subject, it is likely that none of these sources stressed sufficiently the darker side of twin pregnancy, in particular, the high risks associated with MC twinning and the absolute necessity to confirm an accurate and early diagnosis of chorionicity.

Although plans were made regarding delivery and postnatal care, there were none for potential antenatal problems. No diagnosis of impending problems was made by the physician when Claudine began to experience pain (probably related to the hydramnios). Even when she called an obstetrician, she was given an appointment rather than being seen immediately.

The onset of established labor precluded active management of the TTT by, for example, amniocentesis or the effective use of steroids to promote fetal lung maturation. Due to the lack of a second ultrasound examination, almost every complication of twin pregnancy occurred. The emotional costs borne by this family cannot be calculated, although it has probably not been entirely negative. The dollar costs for the twins' healthcare have been high and will continue to be so. However, the prognosis for these boys is not inevitably grim; they may in fact develop relatively well.

Could all of this have been prevented? It is difficult to be certain and easy to be critical after the event. Newer methods for treating TTT have greatly reduced the mortality, but there are no good follow-up studies of morbidity, and many survivors are not neurologically intact. Unfortunately, major advances cannot be made until healthcare providers recognize and react to the high risks inherent in all twin pregnancies and especially to the importance of distinguishing between MC and DC twin outcomes. It is difficult to think of any further efforts Claudine herself could have made to ensure a better pregnancy outcome.

Double twin stillbirth with TTT

Susan thought she had a twin pregnancy. At 13 weeks, she was larger than she had expected to be, and she could already feel fluttering movements. Ultrasonography at this time confirmed her self-diagnosis. Ultrasound examinations were repeated at 17, 22 and 26 weeks, and showed normal fetal growth.

However, at 30 weeks, a different radiologist reported on the ultrasound and, for the first time, commented on the single placental disk and the thin septal membranes, indicative of a likelihood of MC, DA twinning. Further ultrasound examinations at 32 and 34 weeks continued to show normal fetal growth and function, with no hydramnios or oligohydramnios.

Susan felt fine until week 36, when she developed flu-like symptoms. In hospital, she was found to be in early labor, but this ceased by the following morning, when an NST showed minimal cardiac variability. Although Susan and her husband Dale both pleaded for induction of labor, the obstetrician did not consider this to be indicated. The next day, the results of the NSTs were reactive and Susan was sent home. However, she sensed a decrease in fetal movement on the following day, especially of twin A. Eight days after the labor episode, Susan asked for an NST. The nurse had difficulty finding the fetal heart beats, and eventually told Susan to go home. Five days later, ultrasonography showed that both twins had died. The radiologist gave her the news as she lay on the ultrasound table, the cold gel still on her abdomen. (Dale was elsewhere with their son Derek at the time.)

For reasons that are still not clear, Susan, her husband Dale, and her family and friends then had to wait a further 12 h before labor was induced. At 0303 h, their first stillborn daughter, Nicole Janna, was delivered, weighing 7 lb 4 oz (5261 g), and was followed by Kathryn Lesley, who weighed 6 lb 9 oz (4762 g). Both girls were big, beautiful and perfectly formed. Nicole was bruised and edematous whereas Katie was extremely pale with bluish lips and nailbeds. Death had been due to acute TTT (Figure 7.6, page 191).

From the autopsy report, Susan and Dale learned that Nicole had died first, probably from complications of a velamentous cord insertion. Katie had continued to pump her blood through their shared placenta into Nicole and had thereby bled to death. Susan and Dale both believe that their lives have been drastically affected by the death of their twins, who still remain significant to them. Indeed, the following letter was written by them to their lost daughters:

Dear Nicole and Katie,

We were so excited when we learned that our family was going to have twin daughters – a 'perfect' family is how we felt. But all of our hopes and dreams were instantly shattered that September day when the doctor told us you both had died inside Mommy's womb. We became very confused and extremely devastated – our lives have never been the same.

Our shared moments with you both after your delivery will be treasured forever. After Mommy and Grammy bathed you and dressed you, we allowed big brother Derek (2 1/2) to hold you. That had to be one of the most difficult moments for us. The rest of the time Mommy and Daddy cuddled you and talked to you and held you in our arms – 9 whole hours.

We will never forget you, our first-born twin daughters and siblings for brother Derek. You will be in our hearts and part of our lives forever. We are constantly reminded of you and how much we lost when we watch your brother as he continues to grow.

We continue to learn more and more about twin pregnancy, coping with loss and about the continuation of life. Our goal is to educate anyone who will listen to our story, in hopes that other twins and their families will be spared this same death sentence.

Love you forever,
Mommy and Daddy

Susan is pregnant again. She is starting to campaign on behalf of twins and their parents for better understanding of the risks of twin pregnancy and the potentially devastating consequences of MC placentation and TTT. On the basis of how Susan feels now, it is not easy to determine who is less fortunate: the parents whose twins are stillborn, or those whose twins have survived TTT, but must deal with major complications and handicaps.

Critique

Early in the pregnancy, the ultrasound reports failed to mention placentation and / or chorionicity. It is not clear whether the genders of the twins were known. The first truly informative ultrasound report was made at 30 weeks, when the probability of monochorionicity was noted. However, in this case, no evidence of chronic antenatal TTT or significant growth discordance was documented.

The events leading to the fetal death of the first twin are also not clear, but may have been related to a cord complication. Certainly, acute TTT then occurred and resulted in the death of the second twin. This second death would probably not have ensued if the twins had been DC.

It may be strongly argued that labor could have been induced at 36 weeks, as the twins would then have had only a few, if any, significant complications of prematurity at that age. When the mother became aware of decreased fetal movement, the importance of this was not considered in light of tests of fetal wellbeing.

The uniquely unpredictable nature of MC twin pregnancies was clearly in evidence in this case. MC placentation is always associated with potentially life-threatening events and, wherever feasible, MC twins should be removed from such danger whenever they show signs of distress.

Successful antenatal treatment of TTT with intact survival

Jeff and Charlotte had been trying to have a baby for around 2 years when it happened. Pregnancy was diagnosed 6 weeks after the last menstrual period. At 10 weeks, an ultrasound examination showed twins with two sacs. Charlotte went out to the fields to tell Jeff, who was harvesting beans. They sat together in the cab of the combine harvester and daydreamed of twin girls with blue eyes and blonde hair (Figure 7.7 a, page 192).

The first ultrasound examination had indicated that the twins were MC, DA. Their obstetrician knew about TTT, and was aware that not all twin pregnancies resulted in normal twins. Charlotte felt that he was keeping a close watch on this twin pregnancy. Indeed, although she felt perfectly well and had no unusual symptoms at 18 weeks, her obstetrician noted that the fundal height was appropriate for 27 weeks. Therefore, he carried out another ultrasound examination and found evidence of TTT. As a result of this finding, Charlotte underwent fetoscopic laser coagulation (Figure 7.7 b, page 192).

The postnatal growth of the twins is graphically shown in Figure 7.7 c, page 193. The key point of the successful outcome in this case is that the ultrasound examination at 18 weeks showed growth discordance (Figure 7.8 a–f, pages 193–5; and Table 7.1). The obstetrician was no longer able to see the membranous septum, and it was apparent that one twin was surrounded by an excess of fluid (hydramnios) whereas the other twin scarcely had any fluid at all (oligohydramnios) and was 'stuck', and appeared to be dolichocephalic (Figure 7.8 f, page 195). This prompted the obstetrician to be completely frank with Charlotte and Jeff as to the high risk of death for both twins. Various therapeutic options were discussed.

Table 7.1 Ultrasound measurements and calculated gestational age (GA) of Jeff and Charlotte's growth-discordant MC, DA twins with antepartum twin–twin transfusion syndrome at week 18 of gestation

Measurement	Twin A (recipient)	GA (week / day)	Twin B (donor)	GA (week / day)
Abdominal circumference	122 mm	17/4	98 mm	16/0
Femoral length	26 mm	17/4	20 mm	15/5
Head circumference	146 mm	17/3	133 mm	16/3
Biparietal diameter	39 mm	17/4	34 mm	16/1
Estimated fetal body weight	211–221 g	—	141–150 g	—
Calculated GA	—	17/4	—	16/1

Based on unpublished data, courtesy of J. De Lia

The couple decided to seek out Dr Julian De Lia for his assessment, and were also able to obtain helpful and reassuring information from the TTS Foundation in Cleveland. So, from the farmlands of Ohio, they drove to Milwaukee and, on the way, Charlotte read aloud some of the stories of patients who had had laser surgery for TTT. Assessment of the clinical situation was favorable, and the procedure was explained to them by Dr De Lia in detail. Laser surgery was performed 13 days after the diagnosis of TTT. Charlotte was given a general anesthetic, and Jeff waited anxiously near the operating room during the procedure. They stayed in donated hotel rooms.

There were daily clinical checks. Charlotte had a small abdominal incision, which was not painful, and was taking medication to prevent labor. Six days after surgery, the bladder of the donor twin was beginning to fill and fluid was accumulating in her amniotic sac. It was evident that the procedure had been successful.

Before leaving for home, the couple were advised that Charlotte should not do anything physically out of the ordinary to allow the pregnancy to go on for as long as possible. The following $3^1/2$ months seemed endless. They set a goal of 36 weeks and, indeed, succeeded in reaching 37 weeks and 2 days when their obstetrician decided to schedule delivery by Cesarean section.

Christine Marie (recipient) weighed 2730 g at birth and measured 51 cm, and Amanda Renee (donor) weighed 2610 g and measured 46 cm. There is no evidence of any disturbances to brain development or function. Christine (the recipient) has always been larger and is developmentally ahead of Amanda (see Figure 7.7 c).

Critique

Fortune favors the mentally prepared. If every obstetrician had seen or read about at least one case of TTT earlier in his / her career, the problems related to the lack of early detection and treatment of MC placentas and their complications may not be so commonplace. This case shows that TTT can be detected by ultrasound before the mother manifests symptoms. If she arrives in early labor or with ruptured membranes, it is too late for treatment. Speed of decision-making and skilled care are the other components of success.

Familial twinning

It is generally true that families with several pairs of twins are genetically predisposed to DZ twinning. In the course of our respective medical practices, several families have been identified who have more than one pair of MZ twins. Parents and twins themselves are sometimes confused regarding twin zygosity because they expect such twins to be DZ. The family trees and photographs of three families with familial MZ twinning are shown in Figure 7.9 (pages 196–201).

Conjoined twinning

In Part I, Section 3, *Conjoined twinning*, it was pointed out that many types of conjoined twins are not surgically separable, whereas other types may successfully undergo complex staged procedures. Such procedures may achieve satisfactory separation, although some twins may require unequal sharing of organ systems, use of prostheses or the death of one twin to ensure the survival of the other.

To a large extent, these different outcomes depend on the degree to which the organ systems are coalesced or have been disturbed during the formation of new body axes. The following case histories show some of the complexities involved in the planning and decision-taking for conjoined twins who have been separated. Nevertheless, non-separable twins may yet be able to live relatively full lives (see below).

Case 1: Successful separation of minimally conjoined female omphalopagus twins

This set of twins (Figure 7.10a, page 202) were born by vaginal delivery at 36 weeks. Although ultrasound examinations had been performed, the diagnosis was missed because the conjoining was minimal. Consequently, the mutual omphalocele was ruptured, but the other zones of coalescence remained intact. These latter included a urachal bridge and a common large bowel that emptied into the bladder of twin A.

After correction, twin A underwent a colostomy and twin B an ileostomy. Each girl has a complete uterus with tubes and ovaries, but both require further surgery to their genital and urinary structures.

Case 2: Separation of asymmetrical female ischiopagus conjoined twins

These twins (Figure 7.10b, page 202) were born at 37 weeks by Cesarean section as part of a known triplet pregnancy in which the diagnosis of conjoined twinning was not made prenatally. They were asymmetrical in that there were two normal limbs and one less well-formed limb containing partial elements of the two other limbs.

The organs were structured as follows: there were two small bowels as far as the vitellointestinal duct and a common bowel distally, with a single anus; each twin had a single kidney, with the ureters of both running to a single bladder which emptied, via a urethrovaginal fistula, to the vagina of twin B; two complete sets of internal genitalia, and two septate vaginas.

The vestigial limb could not be salvaged. Following skin expansion by pneumoperitoneum, separation was achieved (Figure 7.10c & d, pages 202–3) with the following results: twin A had a single lower limb, a colostomy, a vagina, half of the common bladder and a catheterizable urethral opening made from the appendix; twin B had a single lower limb, a temporary jejunostomy, the anus, a vagina and half of the common bladder with the urethral fistula.

Twin B has progressed well since closure of the jejunostomy and establishment of bowel continuity. Twin A has required revision of the colostomy as well as further surgery to the urinary tract.

Case 3: Separation of symmetrical female ischiopagus conjoined twins

This set of twins had four lower limbs, four kidneys, two bladders (each receiving a ureter from each twin), two septate vaginas, two urethrovaginal fistulae, a common large bowel and one anus. Separation was achieved as shown in Figure 7.10 e (page 203).

Case 4: Separation of asymmetrical male ischiopagus conjoined twins

These twins (Figure 7.10 f, page 203) had a common large bowel, no anus (a rectoperineal fistula was present), a single penis with hypospadias and two scrotums, each containing one testis; each twin had one kidney connected to a large common bladder; there was a single dysplastic kidney. At separation, each twin received half of the bladder and one received the single penis and both testes; he soon died because of tight thoracic closure problems. The other twin underwent construction of female genitalia and a urethrovaginal fistula.

This example illustrates the difficulties in allocating external genitalia in cases of asymmetrical male ischiopagus conjoined twinning.

Case 5: Separation of asymmetrical male ischiopagus conjoined twins

This set of twins (Figure 7.10 g, page 204) was less asymmetrical, each having a penis, although one penis was hypoplastic with hypospadias and severe chordee; there was a common large bowel and one anus. At separation, one twin received the whole bladder and the other had a ureterostomy, which failed to function well. The smaller genitalia lack a prostate gland and an ejaculatory mechanism.

Case 6: Separation of female dicephalic conjoined twins

Apart from one episode of pneumonia (Figure 7.10 h, page 204), these twins were well at the time of assessment for possible surgical separation at age 2 years. The extent of their shared organs (Figure 7.10 i, page 204) are a single urethra, external genitalia, large bowel and anus.

Surgical separation was complex, and the twin on the left did not survive long after the operation. She appeared to have a weaker heart, as is often the case with the left dicephalic twin. The surviving twin has been fitted with a prosthetic left leg and, at the time of writing, has ongoing wound infection and urinary stones.

Case 7: Dicephalic female conjoined twins who have not been separated

The decision not to separate these twins (Figure 7.10 j, page 205) has led their family to adapt to a new lifestyle. Each girl clearly has her own sense of individuality yet, at the same time, is able to cooperate with the other in activities such as tying their shoelaces. There have been no serious health problems, indicating that the girls have independent hearts and lungs.

Their parents wonder how the girls will experience their teenage years, when privacy becomes a priority and when they may not be able to fully experience personal relationships in the same way that other teenagers do. In the meantime, the twins are able to participate in a full range of activities, including swimming and bike-riding, and have virtually no restrictions on what they can achieve.

Mirroring in monozygotic twins

This phenomenon is not well understood, and little systematic research has been carried out on the subject. Mirroring is one of the most puzzling and interesting twin phenomena to both twins and their parents. Much depends on how 'mirroring' is defined. The most marked type of mirroring occurs where one twin had situs solitus (organs in the correct orientation in the thorax and abdomen) and the co-twin has situs inversus (or some variant of it). The true incidence of this condition is unknown. The literature shows no excess of situs inversus among MZ twins nor of MZ twinning among subjects with situs inversus.

The term 'mirroring' in MZ twins usually applies to twins of opposite handedness – right-handed and non-right-handed. In addition, some twin pairs have opposite-sided occipital hair whorls and hair partings (see Figure 7.2). Indeed, opposite handedness suggests that the twins have opposite-sided dominance of cerebral hemispheres, but does this truly constitute mirroring?

First-degree relatives of both DZ and MZ twins exhibit an excess of non-right-handedness. This may suggest that the gene for non-right-handedness is somehow also implicated in the causation of twinning, both DZ and MZ. The opposite expression of handedness in twin pairs could therefore simply represent the differential effect of the gene acting postzygotically on the twins, as is true of many other postzygotic influences (see Part I, Section 1, *Some reasons why monozygotic twins are not identical*). Furthermore, it may be a profound clue to the twinning process itself and, in particular, to any conclusions that might be drawn as to the likely 'plane of cleavage' of MZ twins from the single zygote.

In the case shown in Figure 7.11 (pages 205–6), the apparent mirroring was shown to be more satisfactorily explained as a gradient of changes across both twins. Each child in this pair of MZ twins has fusion of the mandibular (lower jaw) lateral incisor and canine teeth on opposite sides. However, one twin has normal teeth on the other side, whereas the co-twin shows complete absence of the lateral incisor (Figure 7.11 b & c, page 206).

This suggests that there is a gradient of underdevelopment of the lateral incisor tooth from the right side of twin A (complete development) through underdevelopment with fusion (left side of twin A and right side of twin B) to non-development (left side of twin B; Figure 7.11 d, page 206). This phenomenon is different from mirroring, and may be a manifestation of side-to-side gradients that are important in the left / right organization of the body, whether of a singleton or twins and other multiples.

Conclusion

These true stories of the lives of some twins demonstrate the strengths as well as the weaknesses of the status of twins. Without doubt, twins fascinate everyone. Many people go so far as to express the desire to have been a twin, and many women, at least in North America, do not want a routine singleton pregnancy but, instead, wish for something 'special' such as twins or triplets. Unfortunately, neither nature nor the providers of ART services always make these women aware of the true risks (and costs) of multifetal pregnancies. Similarly, routine antenatal obstetric care often fails to consider the different prognoses for MC and DC twins, and the absolute necessity for diagnosis of chorion status in HOMPs.

The increased rates of morbidity and mortality in multifetal pregnancies cannot be significantly lowered until these issues are understood and put into routine practice. In postnatal life, zygosity is also poorly understood. In some instances, zygosity is important for medical reasons, yet many twins as well as their parents lack a secure knowledge of zygosity. We consider knowledge of zygosity to be the special birthright of like-sexed twins. Doubts and concerns about polar-body twinning may thereby be eased. At present, only two centers in the world routinely offer zygosity testing at birth. Twin research continues to be confounded by a tendency to treat twins as a homogeneous whole rather than as discrete groups of varying chorionicity and zygosity, whether naturally or artificially conceived.

A further oversimplification in twin biology is the widespread assumption that MZ twins are 'identical'. There are numerous environmental and genetic reasons why MZ twins are not identical and why, although they may resemble each other closely, they are not 'carbon copies' of each other. Thus, to call MZ twins identical is to confine them in a genetic straitjacket which denies that any other factors influence who they are. (It is also true that some MZ twins are not even genetically identical.) The use of the terms 'identical' and 'fraternal' by healthcare workers, parents and the media is the single factor that most seriously retards a better understanding of twins in terms of obstetric management, childhood development and twin research.

In some ways, our understanding of twinning remains in the Dark Ages. We have few clues as to the cause(s) of MZ twinning and, so far, we have not been able to correlate adverse events in prenatal life with subsequent parameters of postnatal development. We cannot control the medicines prescribed for infertility to avoid superfertility, and our ideas on how to manage TTT are rudimentary. We do not know whether or to what extent mirroring exists in twins. In these and several other matters, we cannot answer many of the questions that twins and their parents most frequently ask about issues affecting their actual day-to-day lives.

If this picture appears overly gloomy, it is intentional in order to dispel any unwarranted complacency regarding the present situation. Too often, twins are lost among the larger issues of prevention and complications of preterm labor, use of advanced imaging technology in prenatal care, studies of nature *vs* nurture and, most recently, whether they can be replaced by human clones.

At this point, it is reasonable to ask how we can improve the current situation. There appear to be two changes that need to be made:

(1) The twinning phenomenon should be considered as a primary entity rather than a significant (or insignificant) component of other larger and more pressing problems; and

(2) Dedicated groups should establish themselves in order to develop the expertise and commitment to deal with the twinning issues that still await clarification. Interested parties would include twins and their families, healthcare professionals and caregivers, funding agencies and researchers. The methods are simple, the epidemiology is not complex and cooperation should lead rapidly to results.

If such changes take place, there will then be grounds for genuine hope that the current epidemic of multifetal pregnancies will receive the attention it deserves. We look forward to the time when the outcomes of HOMPs will be greatly improved. We hope that this book will help to hasten that day when there will be a much deeper understanding of twinning both in practical aspects and in scientific terms.

Selected bibliography

General

Baldwin VJ. *Pathology of Multiple Pregnancy*. New York, Berlin: Springer-Verlag, 1993

Benirschke K, Kaufman P. *Pathology of the Human Placenta*, 3rd edn. New York, Berlin: Springer-Verlag, 1995:719–826

Bryan E. *Twins, Triplets and More: Their Nature, Development and Care*. London: Penguin Books, 1992

Keith LG, Papiernik E, Keith DM, et al., eds. *Multiple Pregnancy: Epidemiology, Gestation and Perinatal Outcome*. New York, London: The Parthenon Publishing Group, 1995

MacGillivray I, Campbell DM, Thompson B, et al., eds. *Twinning and Twins*. Chichester: Wiley & Sons, 1988

Part I, Section I Biology of twins and other multiple pregnancies

Bamforth F, Machin G, Innes M. X-chromosome inactivation is mostly random in placental tissues of female monozygotic twins and triplets. *Am J Med Genet* 1996;61:209–15

Bieber FR, Nance WE, Morton CC, et al. Genetic studies of an acardiac monster: Evidence of polar body twinning in man. *Science* 1981;213:775–7

Botting BJ, Davies IM, Macfarlane AJ. Recent trends in the incidence of multiple births and associated mortality. *Arch Dis Child* 1987;62:941–50

Derom R, Vlietinck RF, Derom C, et al. Zygosity testing at birth: A plea to the obstetrician. *J Perinat Med* 1991; 19(Suppl): 234–40

Derom C, Vlietinck R, Derom R, et al. Increased monozygotic twinning rate after ovulation induction. *Lancet* 1987;i:1236–8

Derom C, Maes H, Derom R, et al. Iatrogenic multiple pregnancies in East Flanders, Belgium. *Fertil Steril* 1993;60:493–6

Fowler MG, Kleinman JC, Keily JL, et al. Double jeopardy: Twin infant mortality in the United States, 1983 and 1984. *Am J Obstet Gynecol* 1991;165:15–22

Goodship J, Carter J, Burn J. X-inactivation patterns in monozygotic and dizygotic female twins. *Am J Med Genet* 1996;61:205–8

Jauniaux E, Elkhaazen N, Leroy F, et al. Clinical and morphological aspects of the vanishing twin phenomenon. *Obstet Gynecol* 1988;72:577–81

Kaplowitz PB, Bodurtha J, Brown J, et al. Monozygotic twins discordant for Ullrich–Turner syndrome. Am J Med Genet 1991;41:78–82

Lupski JR, Garcia CA, Zoghbi HY, et al. Discordance of muscular dystrophy in monozygotic female twins: Evidence supporting asymmetric splitting of the inner cell mass in a manifesting carrier of Duchenne dystrophy. Am J Med Genet 1991;40:354–64

Machin GA. Some causes of genotypic and phenotypic discordance in monozygotic twin pairs. Am J Med Genet 1996;61:216–28

Nance WE. Do twin Lyons have larger spots? [Invited Editorial]. Am J Hum Genet 1990;46:646–8

Perlman E, Stetten G, Tuck-Muller CM, et al. Sexual discordance in monozygotic twins. Am J Med Genet 1990; 37:551–7

Sulak LE, Dodson MG. The vanishing twin: Pathologic confirmation of ultrasound phenomenon. Obstet Gynecol 1986;68:811–5

Winchester B, Young E, Geddes S, et al. Female twin with Hunter disease due to non-random inactivation of the X chromosome: A consequence of twinning. Am J Med Genet 1992;44:834–8

Yokata Y, Akane A, Fujino N, et al. Monozygotic twins of different apparent sex. Am J Med Genet 1994;53:52–5

Part 1, Section 2 Antepartum diagnosis and management of twin pregnancies

Abuhamad AZ, Mari G, Copel JA, et al. Umbilical artery flow velocity waveforms in monoamniotic twins with cord entanglement. Obstet Gynecol 1995;86(4Pt2): 674–7

Alexander JM, Hammond KR, Steinkampf MP. Multifetal reduction of high-order multiple pregnancy: Comparison of obstetrical outcome with nonreduced twin gestations. Fertil Steril 1995;64:1201–3

Benson CB, Doubilet PM, David V. Prognosis of first trimester twin pregnancies: Polychotomous logistic regression analysis. Radiology 1994;192:765–8

Borrell A, Pecarrodona A, Puerto B, et al. Ultrasound diagnostic features of twin reversed arterial perfusion sequence. Prenat Diagn 1990;10:443–8

Bromley B, Benacerraf B. Using the number of yolk sacs to determine amnionicity in early first trimester mono-chorionic twins. J Ultrasound Med 1995;14:415–9

Donnenfeld AE, van de Woestinje T, Craparo F, et al. The normal fetus of an acardiac twin pregnancy: Perinatal management based on echocardiographic and sonographic evaluation. Prenat Diagn 1991;11:235–44

Hertzberg BS, Murtz AB, Choi HY, et al. Significance of membrane thickness in the sonographic evaluation of twin gestations. Am J Radiol 1987;148:151–3

Hill LM, Guzick D, Cheveney P, et al. The sonographic assessment of twin growth discordancy. Obstet Gynecol 1994;84:501–4

Mahony BS, Filly RA, Callen PW. Amnionicity and chorionicity in twin pregnancies: Prediction using ultrasound. Radiology 1985;155:205–29

Monteagudo A, Timor-Tritsch IE, Sharma S. Early and simple determination of chorionic and amniotic type in multifetal gestations in the first fourteen weeks by high-frequency transvaginal ultrasonography. Am J Obstet Gynecol 1994;170:824–9

Patten RM, Mack LA, Nyberg DA, et al. Twin emboliza-tion syndrome: Prenatal sonographic detection and sig-nificance. Radiology 1989;173:685–9

Sharma S, Gray S, Guzman ER, et al. Detection of twin–

twin transfusion syndrome by first trimester ultrasonography. *J Ultrasound Med* 1995;14:635–7

Stiller RJ, Romero R, Pace S, *et al.* Prenatal identification of twin reversed arterial perfusion syndrome in the first trimester. *Am J Obstet Gynecol* 1989;160:1194–6

Tanaka M, Natori M, Ishimoto H, *et al.* Intravascular pancuronium bromide infusion for prenatal diagnosis of twin–twin transfusion syndrome. *Fetal Diagn Ther* 1992; 7:36–40

Watson WJ, Valea FA, Seeds JW. Sonographic evaluation of growth discordance and chorionicity in twin gestation. *Am J Perinatol* 1991;8:342–4

Wood SL, St Onge R, Connor G, *et al.* Evaluation of the twin peak or lambda sign in determining chorionicity in multiple pregnancy. *Obstet Gynecol* 1996;88:6–9

Part 1, Section 3 Understanding the pathology of twin pregnancies

Achiron R, Rosen N, Zakut H. Pathophysiologic mechanism of hydramnios development in twin transfusion syndrome. A case report. *J Reprod Med* 1987;32: 305–8

Annan B, Hutson RC. Double survival despite cord entwinement in monoamniotic twins. Case report. *Br J Obstet Gynaecol* 1990;97:950–1

Bajoria R, Wigglesworth J, Fisk NM. Angioarchitecture of monochorionic placentas in relation to the twin–twin transfusion syndrome. *Am J Obstet Gynecol* 1995;172: 856–63

Bendon RW, Siddiqi T. Clinical pathology conference: Acute twin-to-twin *in utero* transfusion. *Pediatr Pathol* 1989;9:591–8

Benirschke K. The contribution of placental anastomoses to prenatal twin damage. *Hum Pathol* 1992;23:1319–20

Carr SR, Aronson MP, Coustan DR. Survival rates of monoamniotic twins do not decrease after 30 weeks' gestation. *Am J Obstet Gynecol* 1990;163:719–22

Danskin FH, Nielson JP. Twin transfusion syndrome: What are appropriate criteria? *Am J Obstet Gynecol* 1989; 161:365–9

De Lia J, Kuhlmann RS, Harstad TW, *et al.* Fetoscopic laser ablation of placental vessels in severe previable twin–twin transfusion syndrome. *Am J Obstet Gynecol* 1995;172:1202–11

Elliott JP, Urig MA, Clewell WH. Aggressive therapeutic amniocentesis for treatment of twin–twin transfusion syndrome. *Obstet Gynecol* 1991;77:537–40

Fries MH, Goldstein RB, Kilpatrick SJ, *et al.* The role of velamentous cord insertion in the etiology of twin–twin transfusion syndrome. *Obstet Gynecol* 1993;81:569–74

Fusi L, McParland P, Fisk N, *et al.* Twin pregnancy complicated by single intrauterine death: Problems and outcomes with conservative management. *Am J Obstet Gynecol* 1990;97:511–6

Ginsberg NA, Applebaum M, Rabin SA, *et al.* Term birth after midtrimester hysterotomy and selective delivery of an acardiac twin. *Am J Obstet Gynecol* 1992;167:33–7

Gonen R, Hetman E, Asztalos EV, *et al.* The outcome of triplet, quadruplet, and quintuplet pregnancies managed in a perinatal unit: Obsteric, neonatal and follow-up data. *Am J Obstet Gynecol* 1990;162:454–9

Larroche JC, Droulle P, Delezoide AL, *et al.* Brain damage in monozygous twins. *Biol Neonat* 1990;57: 261–78

Lopriore E, Vandenbussche FPHA, Tiersma ESM, *et al.* Twin-to-twin transfusion syndrome: New perspectives. *J Pediatr* 1995;127:675–80

Machin G, Still K, Lalani T. Correlations of placental vascular anatomy and clinical outcomes in 69 monochorionic twin pregnancies. *Am J Med Genet* 1996;61: 229–36

Megory E, Weiner E, Shalev E, *et al.* Pseudomono-amniotic twins with cord entanglement following genetic funipuncture. *Obstet Gynecol* 1991;78:915–7

Nageotte MP, Hurwitz SR, Kaupke CJ, *et al.* Atriopeptin in twin transfusion syndrome. *Obstet Gynecol* 1989;73: 867–70

Quintero RA, Reich H, Puder KS, *et al.* Brief report: Umbilical cord ligation of an acardiac twin by fetoscopy at 19 weeks of gestation. *N Engl J Med* 1994;330:469–71

Reisner DP, Mahony BS, Petty CN, *et al.* Stuck twin syndrome: Outcome in thirty-seven consecutive cases. *Am J Obstet Gynecol* 1993;169:991–5

Robie GF, Payne GG, Morgan MA. Selective delivery of an acardiac acephalic twin. *N Engl J Med* 1989;320:512–3

Saunders NJ, Snijers RJM, Nicolaides KH. Therapeutic amniocentesis in twin–twin transfusion syndrome appearing in the second trimester of pregnancy. *Am J Obstet Gynecol* 1992;166:820–4

Ville Y, Hyett J, Hecher K, *et al.* Preliminary experience with endoscopic laser surgery for severe twin–twin transfusion syndrome. *N Engl J Med* 1995;332:224–7

Wax JR, Blakemore KJ, Blohm P, *et al.* Stuck twin with co-twin nonimmune hydrops: Successful treatment by amniocentesis. *Fetal Diagn Ther* 1991;6:126–31

Weiner CP, Ludomirski A. Diagnosis, pathophysiology, and treatment of chronic twin to twin transfusion. *Fetal Diagn Ther* 1994;9:283–90

Part II, Section 2 How to test twins for zygosity

Akane A, Matsubara K, Shiono H, *et al.* Diagnosis of twin zygosity by hypervariable RFLP markers. *Am J Med Genet* 1991;41:96–8

Azuma C, Kamiura S, Nobunaga T, *et al.* Zygosity determination of multiple pregnancy by deoxyribonucleic acid fingerprints. *Am J Obstet Gynecol* 1989;160:734–6

Derom C, Bakker E, Vlietinck R, *et al.* Zygosity determination in newborn twins using DNA variants. *J Med Genet* 1985;22:279–82

Higgs DR, Wainscoat JS, Flint J, *et al.* Analysis of human alpha-globin gene cluster reveals a highly informative genetic cluster. *Proc Natl Acad Sci USA* 1986;83:5165–9

Hill AVS, Jeffreys AJ. Use of minisatellite DNA probes for determination of twin zygosity at birth. *Lancet* 1985;ii: 1394–5

Kovacs B, Shahbahrami B, Platt LD, *et al.* Molecular genetic prenatal determination of twin zygosity. *Obstet Gynecol* 1988;72:954–6

Nakamura Y, Lappert M, O'Connell P, *et al.* Variable number tandem repeat (VNTR) markers for human gene mapping. *Science* 1987;235:1616–22

Part III Lives of some twins and their parents

Bouchard C, Tremblay A, Despres J-P, *et al.* The response to long-term overfeeding in identical twins. *N Engl J Med* 1990;322:1477–82

Bouchard TJ, Lykken DT, McGue M, *et al.* Sources of human psychological differences: The Minnesota study of twins reared apart. *Science* 1990;250:223–8

Brass LF, Brass LM, Breitner JC, *et al.* A cohort study of twins and cancer. *Cancer Epidemiol Biomarkers Prev* 1995; 4:469–73

Breitner JC. Alzheimer's disease in the National Academy of Sciences – National Research Council Registry of aging twin veterans. III. Detection of cases, longitudinal results, and observations on twin concordance. *Arch Neurol* 1995;52:763–71

Christian JC, Reed T, Carmelli D, *et al.* Self-reported alcohol intake and cognition in aging twins. *J Stud Alcohol* 1995;56:414–6

Coren S. Twinning is associated with an increased risk of left-handedness and inverted writing posture. *Early Hum Dev* 1994;40:23–7

Finkel D, Pedersen N, McGue M. Genetic differences on memory performance in adulthood: Comparison of Minnesota and Swedish twin data. *Psychol Aging* 1995;10: 437–46

Goldberg TE, Torrey EF, Gold JM, *et al.* Genetic risk of neuropsychological impairment in schizophrenia: A study of monozygotic twins discordant and concordant for the disorder. *Schizophr Res* 1995;17:77–84

Graham AJ, Hawkes CH. Twin study using mortality data: A new sampling method. *Int J Epidemiol* 1995;24: 758–62

Gronberg H, Damber L, Damber JE. Studies of genetic factors in prostate cancer in a twin population. *J Urol* 1994;152(5Pt1):1484–7

Harmon C, Rames L. Folie a deux in identical twins. *Hosp Community Psychiatry* 1994;45:1238–9

Hong Y, de Faire U, Heller DA, *et al.* Genetic and environmental influences on blood pressure in elderly twins. *Hypertension* 1994;24:663–70

Keith LG, Machin GA. Zygosity testing: Current status and evolving issues. *J Reprod Med* 1997;42:699–707

McCarren M, Goldberg J, Ramakrishnan V, *et al.* Insomnia in Vietnam era twins: Influence of genes and combat experience. *Sleep* 1994;17:456–61

Partin AW, Page WF, Le BR, *et al.* Concordance rates for benign prostatic disease among twins suggest hereditary influence. *Urology* 1994;44:646–50

Sokol DK, Moore CA, Rose RJ, *et al.* Intrapair differences in personality and cognitive ability among young monozygotic twins distinguished by chorion type. *Behav Genet* 1995;25:457–66

Steinmetz H, Herzog A, Schlaug G, *et al.* Brain (A) symmetry in monozygotic twins. *Cereb Cortex* 1995;5: 296–300

Stunkard AJ, Harris JR, Pedersen NL, *et al.* The body-mass index of twins who have been reared apart. *N Engl J Med* 1990;322:1483–7

Sumethkul V, Jirasiritham S, Sura T, *et al.* Renal transplantation between identical twins: The application of reciprocal full-thickness skin grafts as a guideline for antirejection therapy. *Transpl Proc* 1994;26:2141–2

Yokoyama Y, Shimizu T, Hayakawa K. Prevalence of cerebral palsy in twins, triplets and quadruplets. *Int J Epidemiol* 1995;24:943–8

Part IV MULTIPLE PREGNANCY ILLUSTRATED

List of illustrations

Part I, Section 3 Understanding the pathology of twin pregnancies

Facing page Hauser mother with her DZ twins (lower left); Specimen obtained during surgery for tubal ectopic pregnancy shows MC, DA MZ twin embryos, each within its own amniotic sac (upper right). One of the two yolk sacs can also be seen

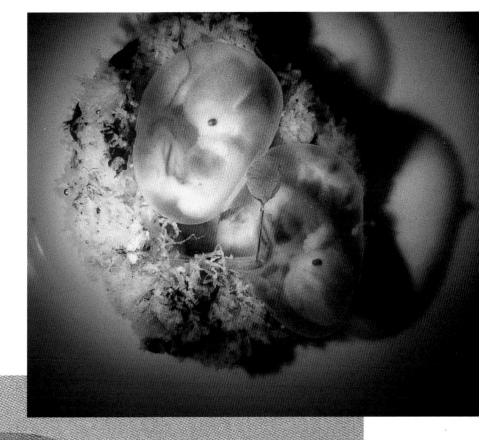

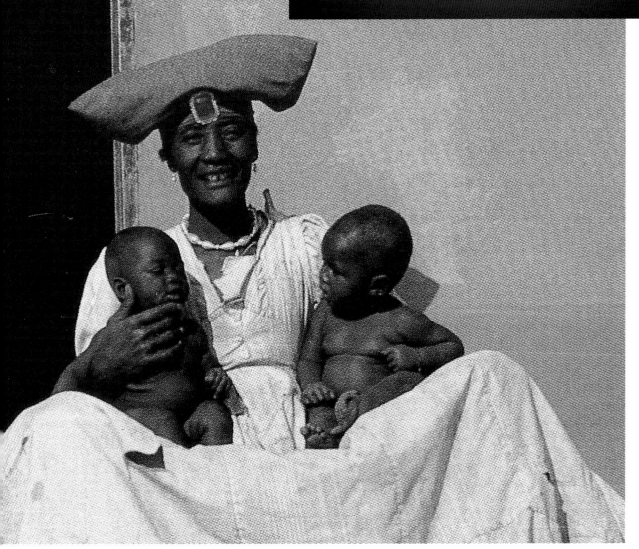

Part I, Section I Biology of twins and other multiple pregnancies

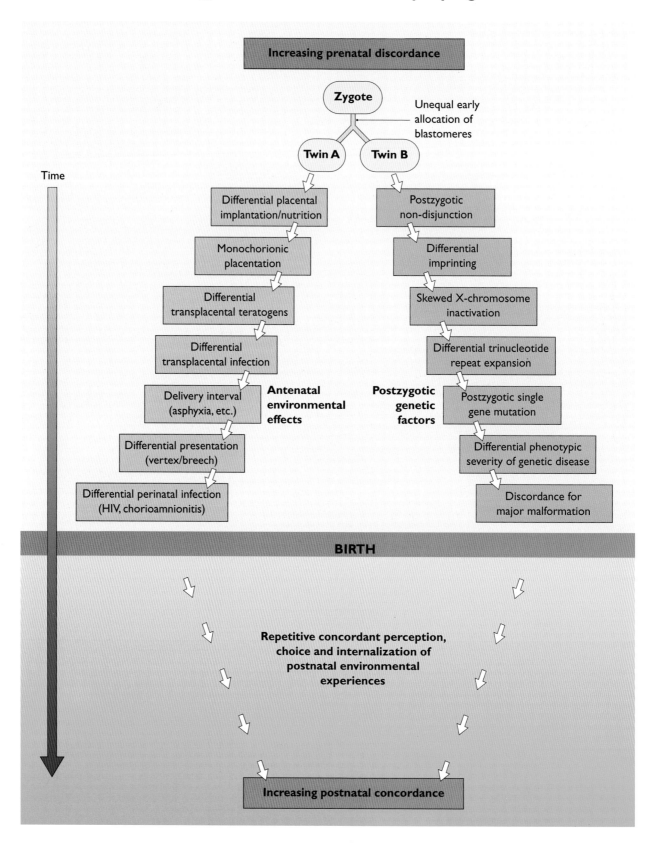

Figure 1.1 Principal mechanisms by which genotype and environment cause discordant phenotypes in monozygotic (MZ) twin pairs:

(1) *Early embryogenesis in MZ twin formation.* From X-chromosome inactivation studies (different clone sizes), there is good evidence that unequal numbers of embryonic cells may be allocated to the twins from the original zygote or inner cell mass. Some major processes in early embryogenesis may depend on timing, in that a 'critical mass' of cells needs to be accumulated before that process can be initiated. Such effects could therefore account for some cases of vanishing twins, fetus papyraceus, twin reversed arterial perfusion (TRAP), twin–twin transfusion (TTT) and discordance for major malformations as well as for growth.

(2) *Postzygotic genetic mechanisms.* Postzygotic chromosomal non-disjunction is the cause of chromosomal mosaicism in singletons. In MZ twinning, it may result in one twin being chromosomally abnormal (for example, with Down or Turner syndrome) whereas the other twin is normal. In addition, an apparently normal co-twin to a trisomic twin may have uniparental disomy.

Postzygotic single-gene mutations have been proven to cause discordance for clinical expression of a single-gene disease in a given MZ twin pair (see also imprinting and trinucleotide repeat expansion below). Discordant mutations in segments of DNA that are not within genes are known to occur in the postzygotic period in MZ twins. Such mutations call into question one of the 'gold standards' for zygosity testing – analysis of multiple DNA segments for any recognizable differences considered to identify the twins as DZ.

The process of gene imprinting occurs in the postzygotic period and may result in MZ twins who are discordant for imprinted single-gene diseases, such as Beckwith–Wiedemann syndrome.

Skewed X-chromosome inactivation is seen in some female MZ twin pairs and may be sufficiently severe as to cause clinical expression of an X-linked disease (such as Duchenne muscular dystrophy) in one female MZ twin, but not the other.

For known genetic diseases, including single-gene diseases, such as tuberous sclerosis and neuro-fibromatosis, and chromosomal trisomies, MZ twin pairs may show discordant degrees of severity of clinical expression. It is not clear whether this may be due to mosaicism.

Differential trinucleotide repeat expansion has been observed in MZ twins, which is a further suggestion that various kinds of DNA tests may not be infallible in zygosity testing.

MZ twins are frequently discordant for major malformations, such as neural tube defects.

(3) *Antenatal and perinatal environmental influences.* Growth discordance is common in MZ and dizygotic (DZ) twins, and may reflect the fact that only one of the dichorionic (DC) placentas is optimally implanted posterosuperiorly. This is one of the ways in which the intrauterine environment is not the same for each twin.

Monochorionic (MC) placentation (two-thirds of MZ twins) may cause marked environmental differences between pairs of MZ twins, including TTT, TRAP and severe growth discordance. Some types of congenital heart disease are caused by abnormal blood flow during embryonic life. In twins, such abnormalities may be caused by the connections between the twin fetal circulations of MC twins. The lifelong sequelae of these effects are largely unknown.

Doses of transplacental teratogens delivered to a twin pair are not necessarily equal, perhaps because of a more or less favorable implantation of the DC placentas. Similarly, in the presence of TTT, an MC twin may transfuse teratogen into the other.

Transport of transplacental infectious agents (principally viruses) is also not necessarily equal.

The delivery interval may adversely affect pH and blood gases in the second-born twin who, in any event, is often the smaller. In MC twins, acute perinatal TTT may arise during this interval. These variables are seldom considered in twin studies.

Differing presentations during delivery may cause lifelong differences in cerebral function.

Ascending infection (chorioamnionitis) more commonly affects the lower gestation sac. Some cases of 'congenital' HIV infection are acquired from maternal tissues and/or secretions during passage through the birth canal. In twin births, the first-born twin is more often affected than is the second

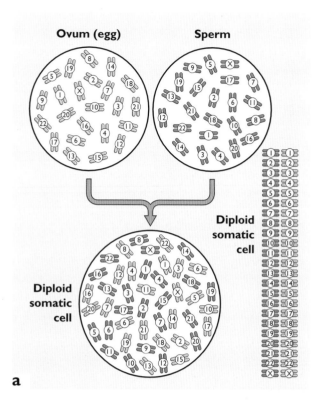

a

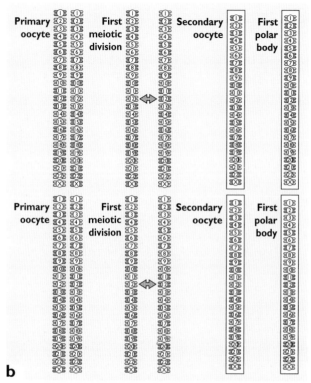

b

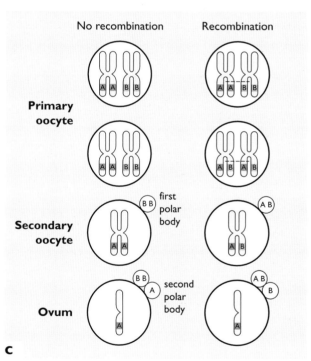

c

Figure 1.2 Polar-body twins do not have similar maternal genetic contributions:

(a) Diploid cells, including the fertilized egg (zygote), contain 23 pairs of homologous chromosomes, in each of which one chromosome is of maternal origin and the other is of paternal origin.

(b) During oogenesis, the homologous chromosomes pair up, but in random arrays of both maternally and paternally derived chromosomes. Each oocyte and ovum therefore has a different chromosomal constitution from all the others whether produced in the same or in subsequent cycles. Thus, in two such arrays of chromosomes, each secondary oocyte has exactly the opposite (reciprocal) array of chromosomes as has its corresponding first polar body.

(c) Each of the allelic genes of a homologous chromosome pair is segregated at first meiosis. However, this effect may be modified by recombination (crossover), resulting in new chromosomal arrays of alleles that did not exist before meiotic division. Thus, in a woman with blood type AB, for example, if no crossover occurs between the locus and centromere at first meiosis, the ovum and first polar body will have reciprocal alleles, but the ovum and second polar body will carry the same allele. If

net crossover does occur, then neither polar body will carry the same allele as the ovum. Considering the total number of alleles for all 23 chromosome pairs, it is highly unlikely that an ovum and its corresponding polar bodies will be genetically similar

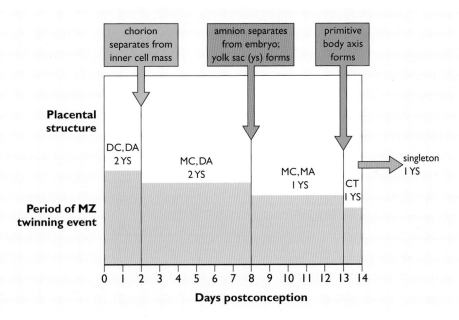

Figure 1.3 Timing of MZ twinning events is related to placental anatomy: The earlier the event, the less closely apposed are the twin pair, and the more physiologically independent they will be. Conjoined twins (CT) are the result of varying degrees of overlapping body plans laid down within one ectoderm

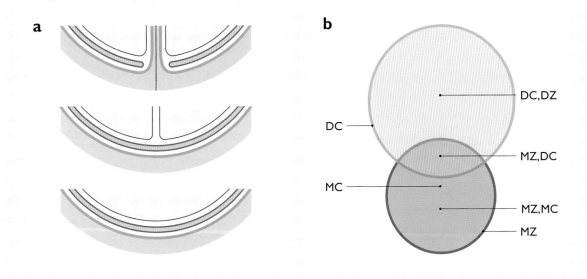

Figure 1.4 Relationship between zygosity and chorionicity:

(a) Fused DC (upper), MC, DA (middle) and MC, MA (lower): DC twins may be DZ or MZ. The DC septum prevents vascular communication (red). MC, DA and MC, MA placentas are always MZ and usually have vascular anastomoses;

(b) All MC twins are MZ, but not all MZ twins are MC. Likewise, all DZ twins are DC, but not all DC twins are DZ as one-third of MZ twins are DC

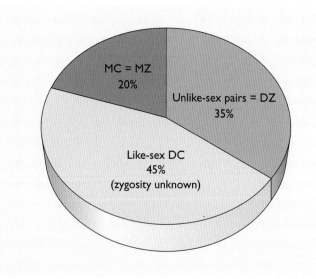

Figure 1.5 Zygosity in relation to gender and chorion status: Zygosity of twins can be determined easily in around 55% of cases. MC twins are MZ and unlike-sex pairs are DZ, but DC like-sexed twins (45%) are not all DZ and, thus, zygosity testing is required for a definitive diagnosis

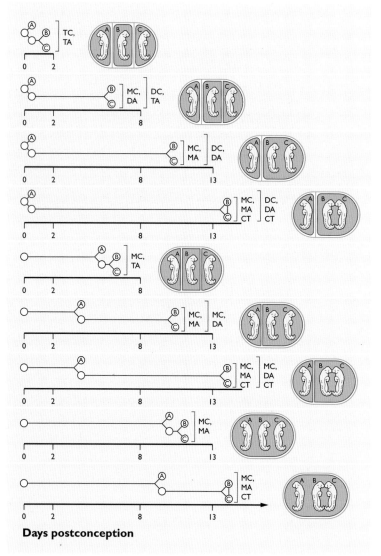

Figure 1.6 Timing of successive twinning events in MZ triplets: These multiples exhibit various combinations of DC, MC, DA and MA placentations as well as conjoined twinning (CT), probably as a result of different timings of twinning events

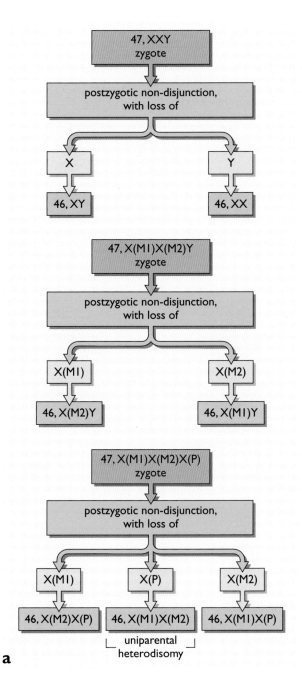

uniparental
heterodisomy

a

Figure 1.7 (a) Hypothetical mechanisms for the production of chromosomally normal MZ twin pairs with different chromosome constitutions:

(upper) It is theoretically possible for a 47,XXY zygote to lose different sex chromosomes in two postzygotic non-disjunctional events, resulting in chromosomally normal female and male MZ twins;

(middle) A 47,XXY zygote could also give rise to MZ male twins of different chromosomal constitutions, depending on which maternal X chromosome was inherited. By this mechanism, a pair of MZ male twins may be discordant for an X-linked disease for which the mother is an obligate carrier;

(lower) Likewise, a 47,XXX zygote could give rise to three MZ female pairs who are not genetically identical because of differences in the parental origins of their X chromosomes. One of these females would show the effects of uniparental disomy.

None of the three above-mentioned events has yet been reported.

(b) Trisomic zygotes that revert to euploid disomy (with or without mosaicism) may have unpredictable consequences, particularly if the non-disjunction occurs at second meiosis, resulting in uniparental isodisomy. The example here shows segregation of an autosomal-recessive mutant allele during spermatogenesis in a heterozygous (unaffected) male (1); the mother is homozygous normal for the gene. The resulting trisomic zygote has two copies of the mutant gene, and there are two possible patterns of postzygotic compensatory loss of the extra chromosome (2): one produces a heterozygous carrier; the other results in a homozygous affected cell line. If these two events were to occur in the context of MZ twinning, the twin pair could be discordant for expression of an autosomal-recessive disease

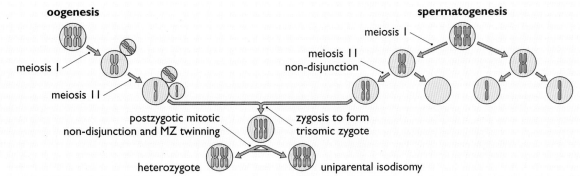

b

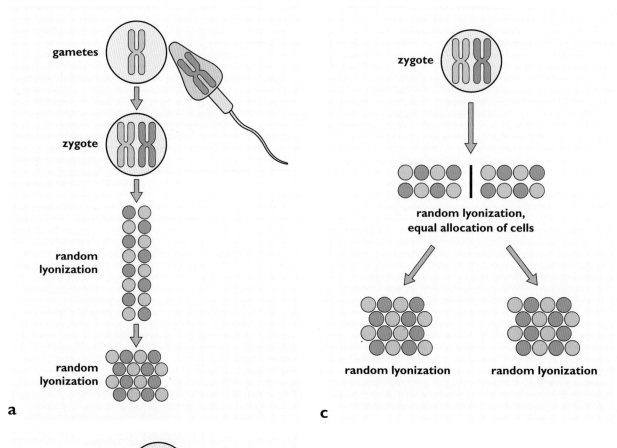

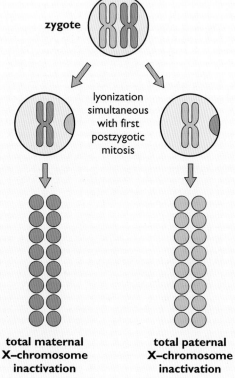

Figure 1.8 Possible patterns of X-chromosome inactivation in female MZ twin pairs:

(a) Singleton females usually show a random or non-skewed pattern of X-chromosome inactivation in all tissues;

(b) If X-chromosome inactivation occured immediately after conception at the time of first postzygotic mitosis, all female MZ twin pairs would show totally oppositely skewed X-chromosome inactivation. (This pattern has never been observed.);

(c) If X-chromosome inactivation is random throughout the early cell mass, both MZ twins will show random inactivation. (This is the most common pattern.);

(d) If X-chromosome inactivation is random throughout the early cell mass, reciprocal patterns

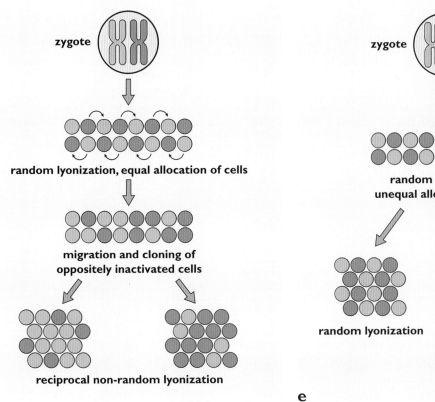

random lyonization, equal allocation of cells

migration and cloning of
oppositely inactivated cells

reciprocal non-random lyonization

d

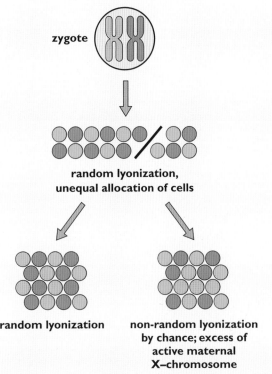

random lyonization,
unequal allocation of cells

random lyonization

non-random lyonization
by chance; excess of
active maternal
X–chromosome

e

of X-chromosome inactivation could develop in different zones by processes of 'recognition', 'aggregation' and 'migration' of cells of similar X-chromosome inactivation status. It has been postulated that this cloning effect may be the cause of some twinning events in MZ female twins. (This pattern has been seen in some MZ pairs.);

(e & f) If X-chromosome inactivation is random throughout the early cell mass, an unequal allocation of numbers of cells to each of the twins may, by chance, result in skewed X-chromosome inactivation in the smaller mass whereas the larger mass will maintain random inactivation. (This pattern has been seen in some MZ pairs which also show other confirmatory evidence that different numbers of cells have contributed to the formation of each twin embryo.)

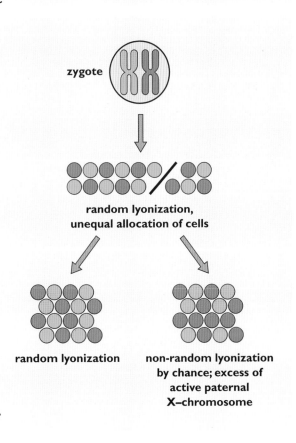

random lyonization,
unequal allocation of cells

random lyonization

non-random lyonization
by chance; excess of
active paternal
X–chromosome

f

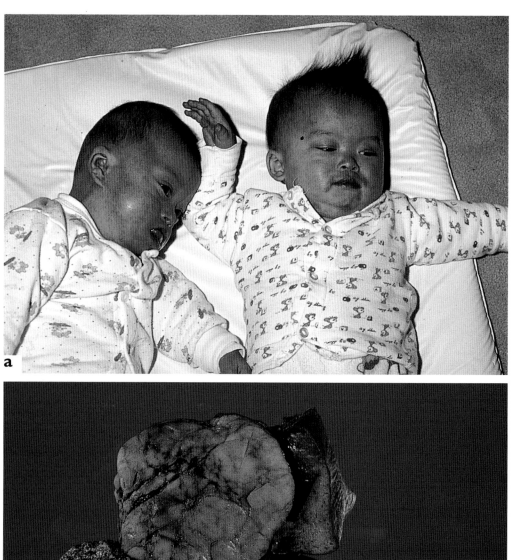

Figure 1.9 MZ twins discordant for Beckwith–Wiedemann syndrome:

(a) These twins are MZ by DNA variable number tandem repeat (VNTR) testing. The twin on the left has Beckwith–Wiedemann syndrome whereas his co-twin appears normal;

(b) At 1 year of age, the affected twin developed a hepatoblastoma, which was resected.

This case reinforces the fact that imprinting phenomena are, at least in part, postzygotic and that the ratios may vary between each MZ twin of a pair

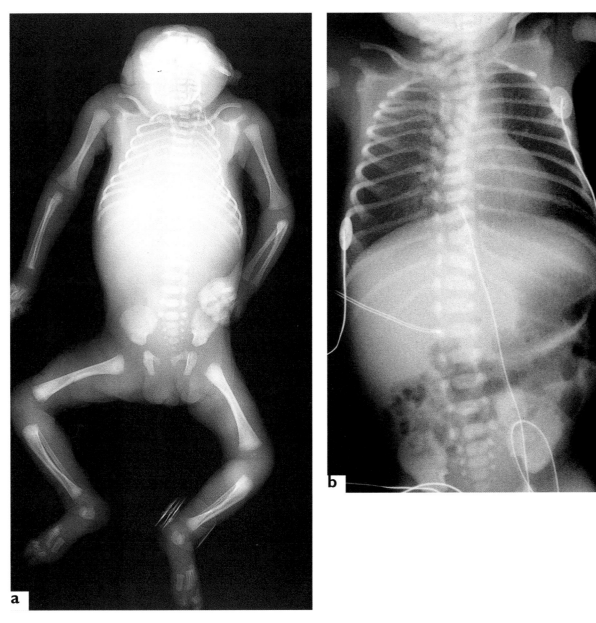

Figure 1.10 MZ twins may often be discordant for major malformations, leading to the erroneous assumption that they are DZ:

(a) These twins were MC. This twin had classic anencephaly with absence of calvarial bones;

(b) The surviving twin has multiple thoracic hemivertebrae, but no other malformations. This finding suggests that anencephaly and hemivertebrae are caused by the same mechanism, probably malformation of the notochord

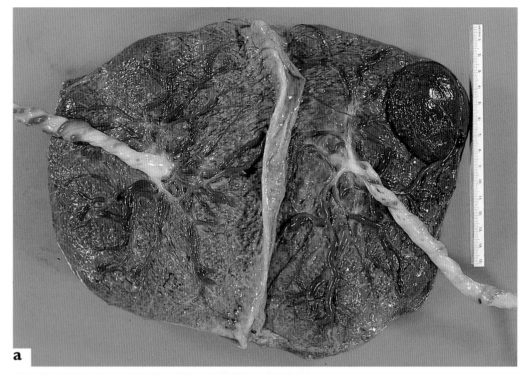

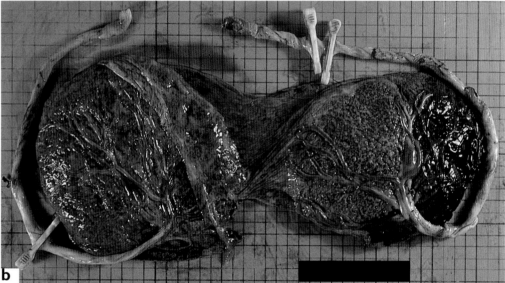

Figure 1.11 Patterns of placentation in twin pairs:

(a & b) In DC twins (whether DZ or MZ), the chorion invests each gestation sac and, thus, is present in the septal membranes. Two distinct chorial layers are not always detectable by ultrasound, especially in later gestation, but the septum is substantial in thickness − > 2 mm. The placental disks may be fused (a) or separate (b);

(c) In MC twins, the entire gestation sac is invested by the single chorion, which therefore cannot participate in the structure of the septal membranes. When the gestation is MC, DA, each twin has its own amniotic cavity and the septum consists of only two layers of amnion. This septum is thin and is often difficult to detect by ultrasound. Vascular anastomoses are frequently present;

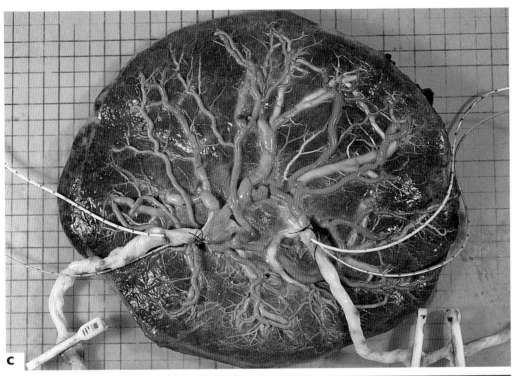

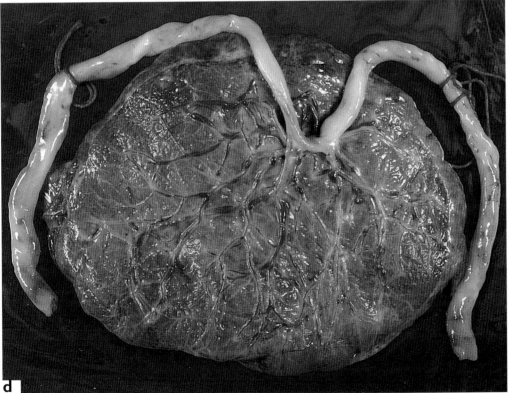

(d) In MC, MA twins, the entire gestation is invested by the single chorion and amnion, and no septum is present. This rare twin placental type most closely resembles a singleton placenta. Note the forked (conjoined) cord in this example, an indication of the closeness in timing to conjoined twinning;

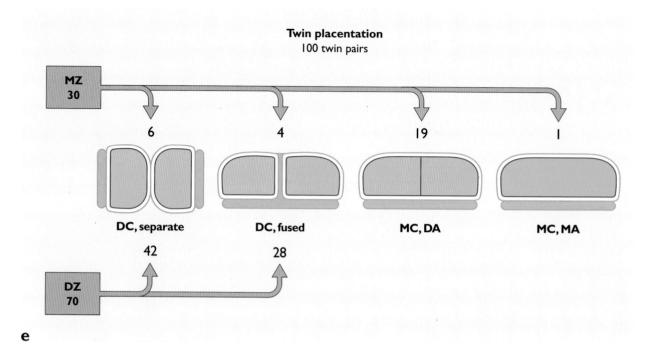

e

f

Figure 1.11 continued
   (e) Relationships between zygosity and chorionicity per 100 spontaneously conceived twin pairs;
   (f) A fused DC placenta, an MC, DA placenta and an MC, MA placenta

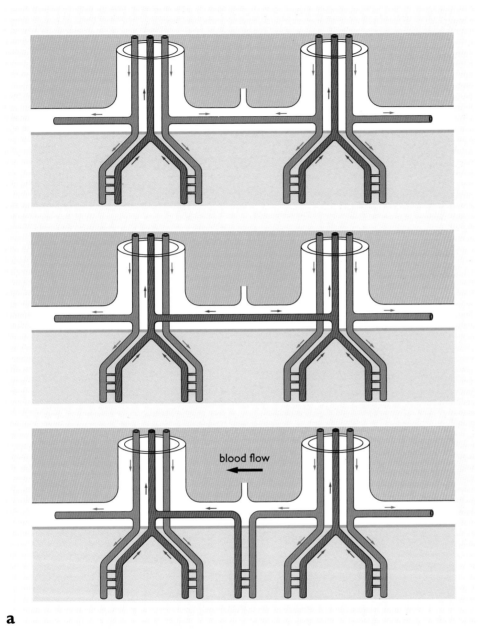

a

Figure 1.12 Patterns of vascular anastomosis in MC placentas:

(a, upper) An a↔a anastomosis runs above the chorionic plate and below the amnion between the insertions of the two umbilical cords. There may be no net flow in this vessel unless there are significant differences between the cardiac outputs of the twins. These anastomoses are commonly seen in MC placentas and cause the arterial systems of the twins to function virtually as one physiological entity;

(a, middle) A v↔v anastomosis runs above the chorionic plate between the insertions of the two umbilical cords. Although there is not necessarily any flow in this connecting vessel, large volumes of blood may rapidly shift if there are even small changes in hemodynamics between the twins. As the v↔v type of anastomosis is rare in MC placentas, the venous systems of twins usually function separately;

(a, lower) An a→v anastomosis in the parenchyma allows the afferent (arterial) vessel to meet the efferent (venous) vessel 'nose-to-nose' above the chorionic plate, but there is no actual connection on the surface. Transfusion of blood is across the villous capillaries deep in the parenchyma;

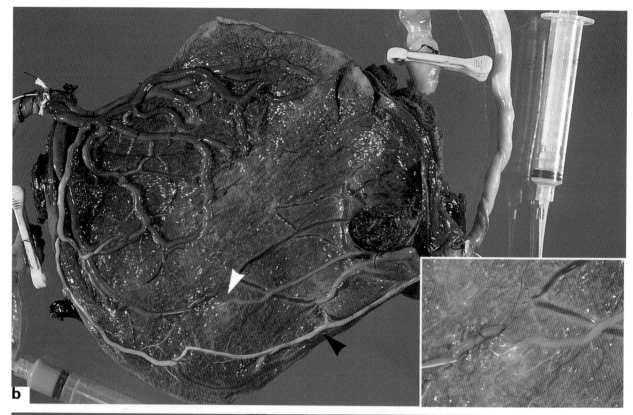

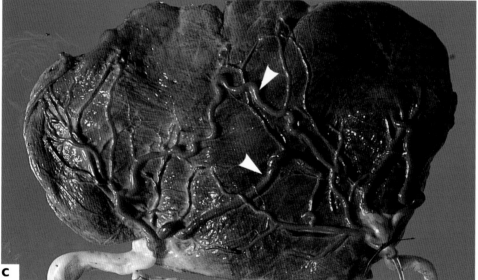

Figure 1.12 continued

(b) Vascular injection shows a superficial a↔a anastomosis (yellow; black arrow) and an a→v anastomosis (white arrow; see inset), which represents inappropriate drainage of a perfusion zone. (Inset) The afferent artery (yellow) is supplied by one twin, but the efferent vein (green) returns to the other twin on the left;

(c) Vascular injection shows a v↔v connection (blue; arrow) and an a↔a anastomosis (red; arrow).

These anastomoses vary in frequency, and may be single, multiple or in combination. A combination of a↔a and a→v anastomoses is the most frequent pattern seen in MC placentas

Part I, Section 2 Antepartum diagnosis and management of twin pregnancies

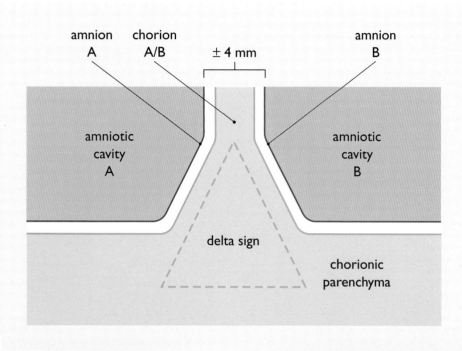

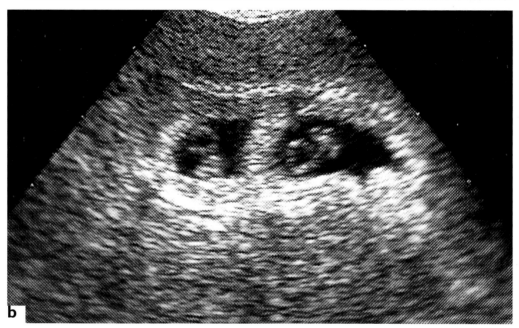

Figure 2.1 DC, DA septum:

(a) Each gestation sac is surrounded by a chorion and an amnion, and both are present in the septum. Two distinct layers of chorion are rarely distinguishable. Where the membranous chorion meets the placental surface, the two chorionic layers diverge to create the 'delta sign'. The septum is substantial, around 4 mm in thickness, and is usually easily visualized;

(b) Typical ultrasound DC septal appearances at 6 weeks of gestation;

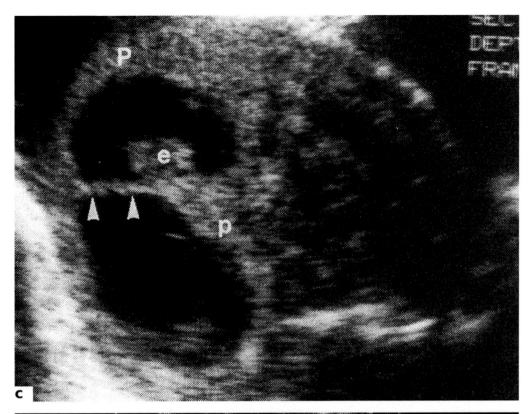

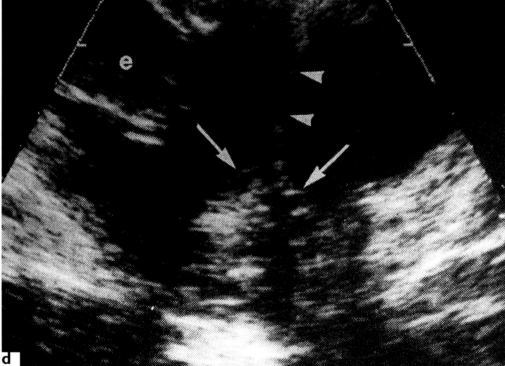

Figure 2.1 continued
    (c) Typical ultrasound DC appearances of a thick membrane (arrows) and delta sign;
    (d) Ultrasound appearances of a thinner DC membrane (arrowheads) and delta sign (long arrows);

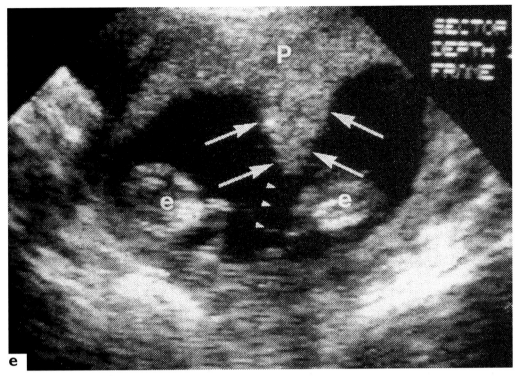

(e) Ultrasonogram showing a well-developed delta sign (long arrows), but the DC membrane is thin (arrowheads)

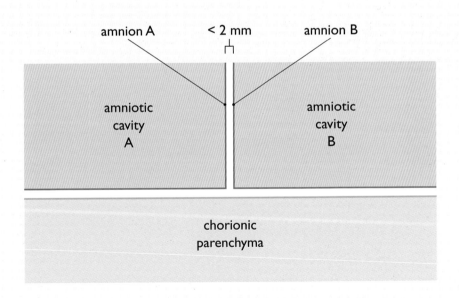

Figure 2.2 MC, DA twin placental septum:

(a) The whole pregnancy is surrounded by a single chorionic sac. Therefore, the chorion does not participate in the formation of the septum, which consists of only two thin layers of amnion. The septum is rather thin, <2 mm thick, and is often difficult to visualize by ultrasound;

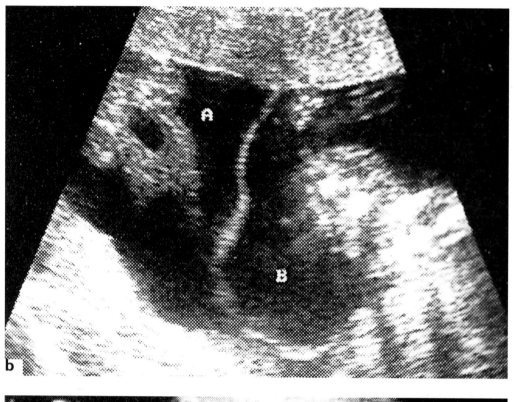

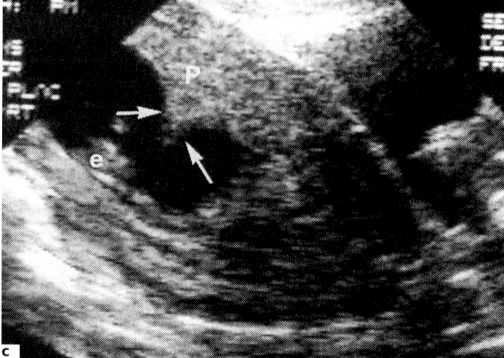

Figure 2.2 continued

(b) Ultrasonogram of an MC,DA septum during the first trimester shows a thin septum which lacks a delta sign;

(c) Ultrasonogram of an MC ,DA septum showing a false-positive delta sign (arrows);

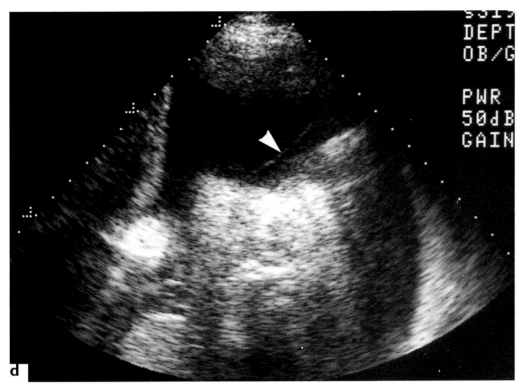

(d) Ultrasonogram of a further MC, DA septum shows a wispy structure running parallel to the placental surface and apparently extending only part of the way across the gestational sac

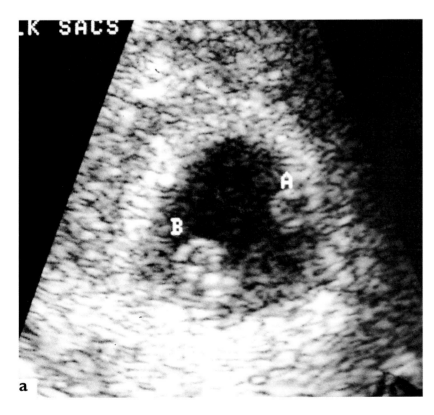

Figure 2.3 Exclusion of MC, MA twins:

(a) Ultrasonogram showing the presence of two yolk sacs (A and B), which excludes MC, MA placentation, even though the septum cannot be seen;

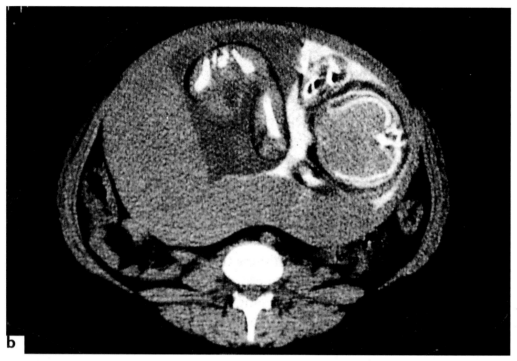

Figure 2.3 continued
(b) On CT examination, MC, MA placentation can be excluded by injection of contrast at one pole of the gestational sac which clearly reveals the outline of one of the two sacs, thereby implying the presence of a septum

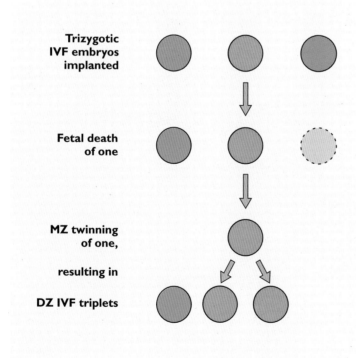

Trizygotic IVF embryos implanted

Fetal death of one

MZ twinning of one,

resulting in

DZ IVF triplets

Figure 2.4 MZ twins among IVF multiple embryos: A combination of embryonic death and MZ twinning may result in apparently anomalous zygosity in multiple pregnancy. In a hypothetical case, three embryos are implanted. One of them 'vanishes' while one of the survivors splits into MZ twins. Although the resultant number of fetuses is the same as the number of implanted embryos, it is clearly wrong to assume trizygosity

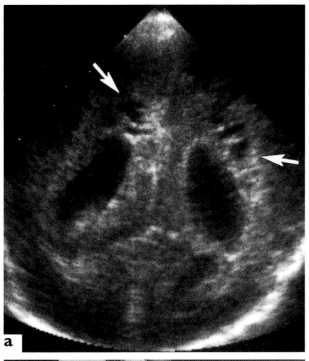

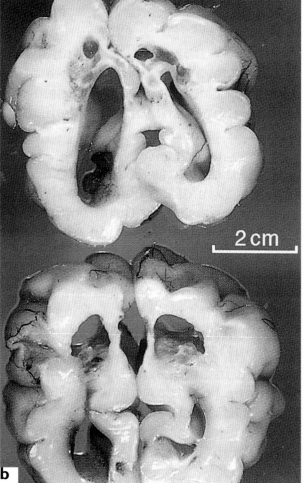

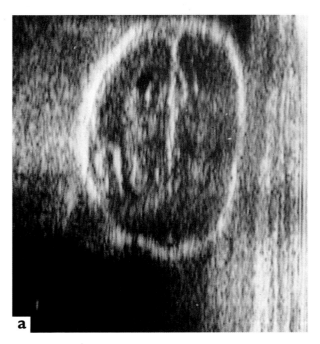

Figure 2.5 Organ infarction following the death of one MC twin:

(a) Neurosonogram showing porencephaly and periventricular leukomalacia (arrowed) in a newborn twin survivor;

(b) Coronal sections of the same brain show ventriculomegaly, cystic encephalomalacia and periventricular leukomalacia

Figure 2.6 Vascular complications in MC twins (TTT and TRAP): Discordance and patterns of vascular flow in antenatal TTT:

(a) Ultrasonogram showing the dolichocephalic head of the 'stuck' twin compressed against the placental surface. For this reason, abdominal circumference and diameter rather than head measurements should be used for assessing growth discordance;

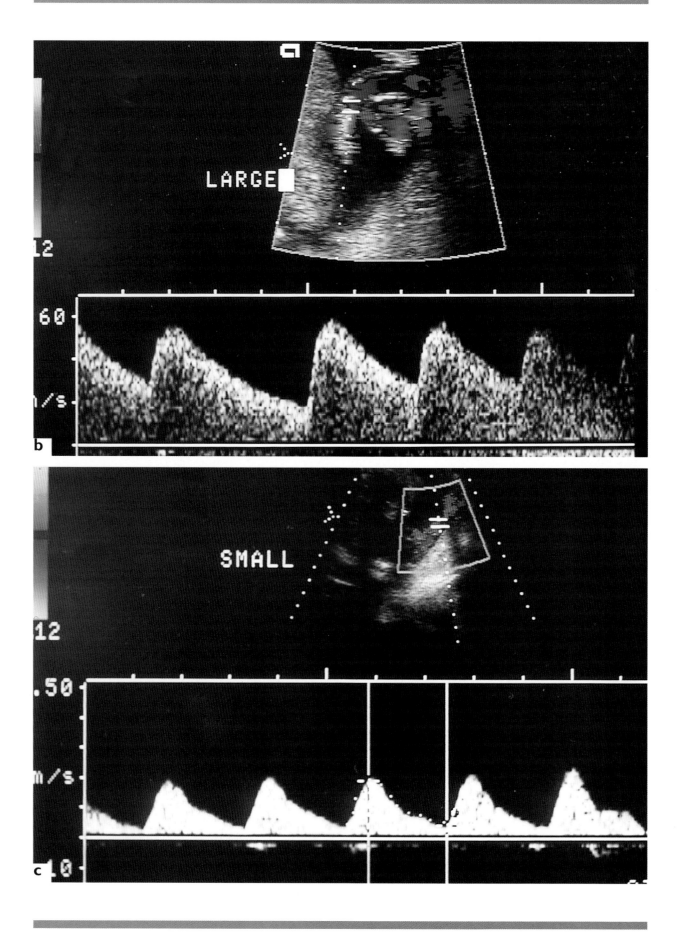

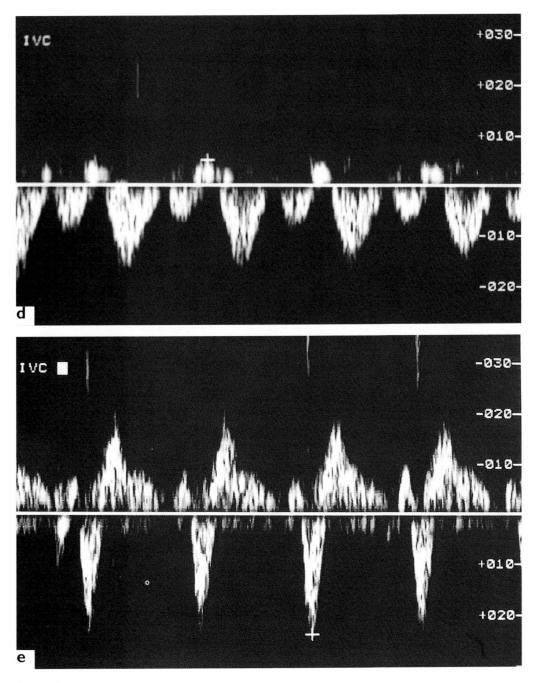

Figure 2.6 continued

(b) Where the umbilical cord of the recipient is large and has marked venous dilatation, CDI shows high peak-systolic and end-diastolic umbilical arterial waveforms;

(c) Where the cord of the donor is small, CDI shows low peak-systolic and end-diastolic arterial flow;

(d) Doppler ultrasonogram of the donor shows a normal triphasic IVC waveform pattern, with a peak velocity of 0.05 m/s;

(e) Doppler ultrasonogram of the recipient shows an elevated IVC peak velocity (0.24 m/s) during atrial contraction, which is characteristic of increased right ventricular pressure with tricuspid regurgitation

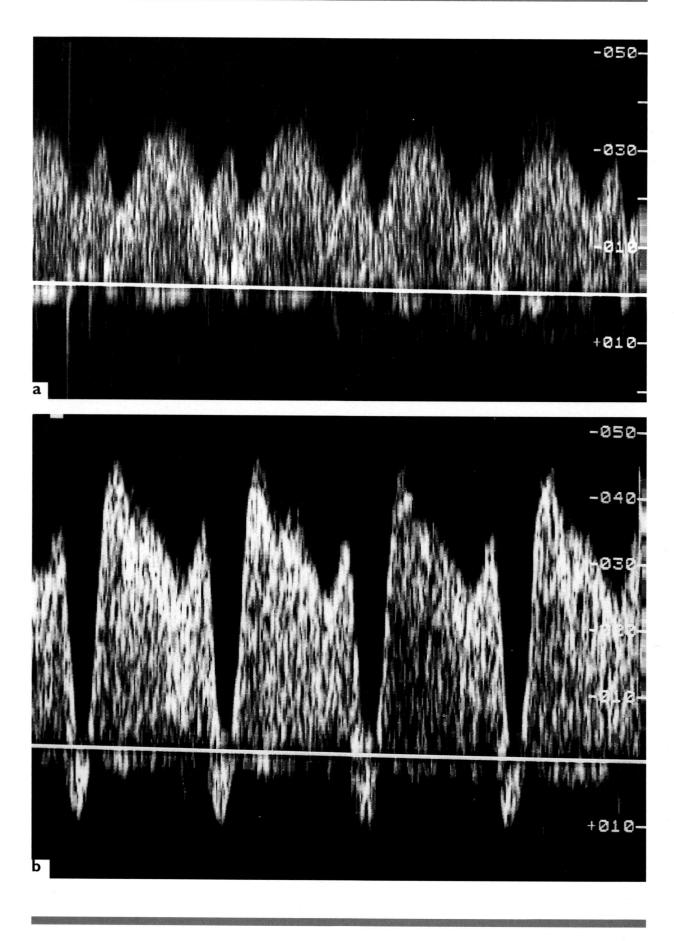

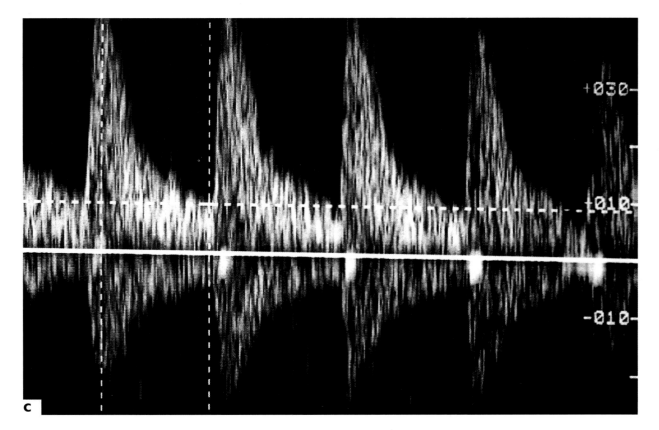

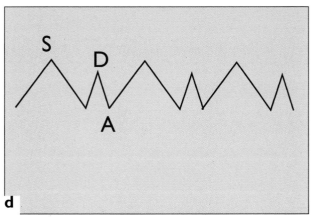

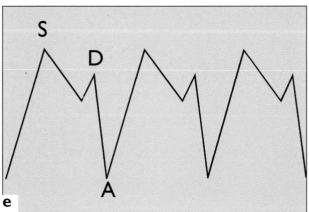

Figure 2.7 Vascular complications in MC twins (TTT and TRAP): Patterns of flow in the ductus venosus:

(a) Doppler ultrasonogram of the ductus venosus of the donor shows a normal triphasic antegrade pattern, with maximum peak velocity during systole (S), a lesser peak in diastole (D) and minimum velocity during atrial contraction (A; see diagram of trace d);

(b) Doppler ultrasonogram of the ductus venosus of the recipient shows retrograde flow during atrial contraction (A; see diagram of trace e);

(c) Doppler ultrasonogram of middle cerebral artery blood flow of the donor in antepartum TTT shows an S:D ratio of 5.13:1;

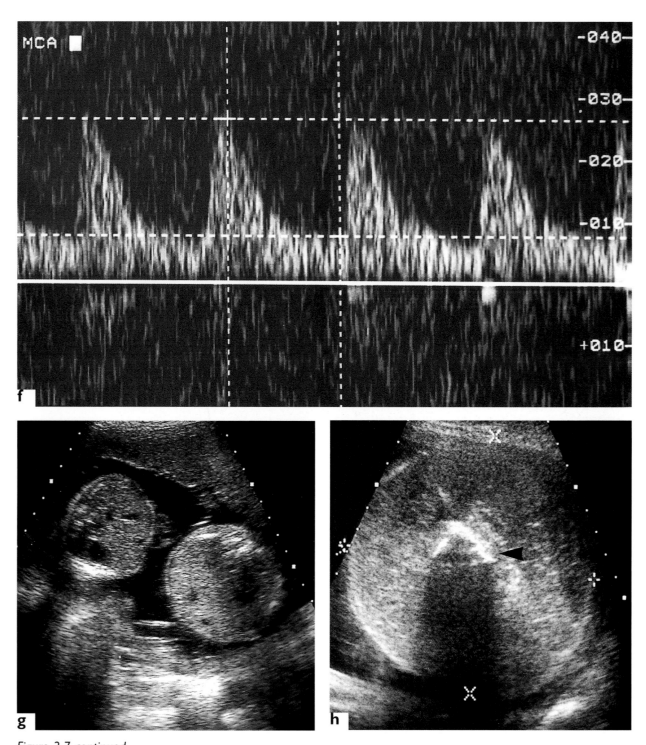

Figure 2.7 continued

(f) Doppler ultrasonogram of middle cerebral artery blood flow of the recipient shows an S : D ratio of only 3.60 : 1;

(g) Ultrasonogram showing transverse views of the abdomens of both donor (to the left) and recipient (to the right) in antenatal TTT;

(h) Ultrasonogram showing transverse view of the torso of the acardiac twin in TRAP. There is a primitive vertebra (arrow), but no evidence of abdominal viscera

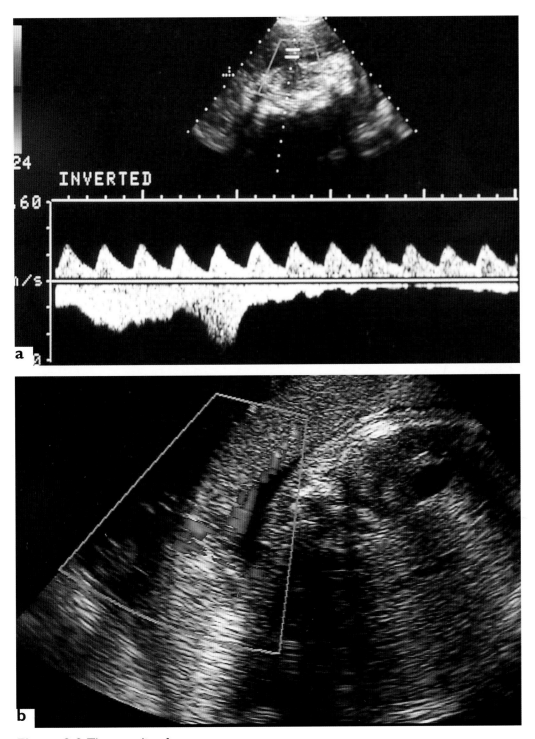

Figure 2.8 The acardiac fetus:

(a) CDI showing the two-vessel cord of an acardiac twin. The venous flow rates are modulated by the breathing pattern of the pump twin. The acardiac twin may be considered a 'parasite' of the pump twin;

(b) CDI showing the vessels exiting from the cord of the acardiac twin to be large, superficial, communicating vessels to the pump twin. There is also vascular flow in the maternal spiral arteries

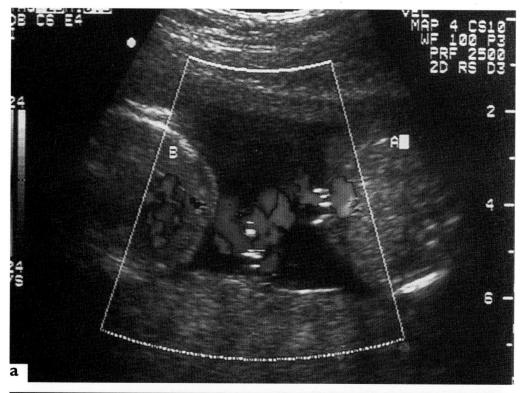

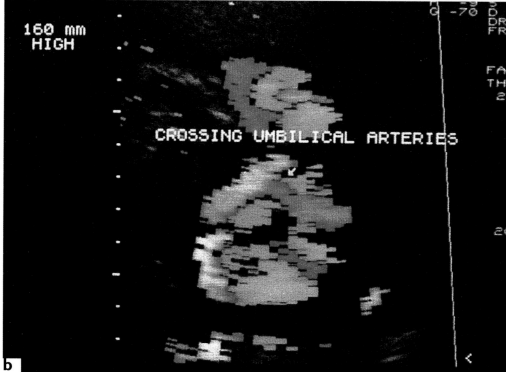

Figure 2.9 Cord entanglement in MC, MA twins:

(a) CDI shows complex braiding with overlapping vessels, appearances suggestive of 'branching';

(b) CDI shows two crossing umbilical arteries and two different flow rates;

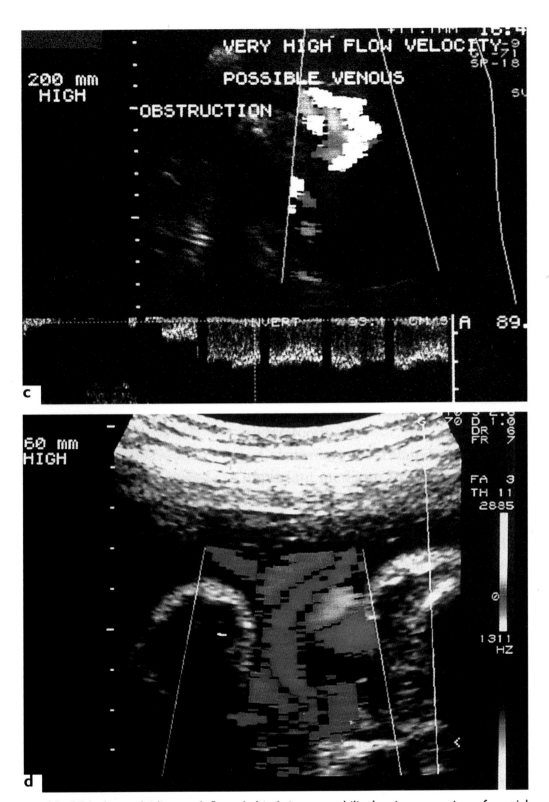

(c) CDI shows high-speed flow (white) in an umbilical vein suggestive of partial obstruction by knots;

(d) CDI shows two crossing umbilical veins (blue);

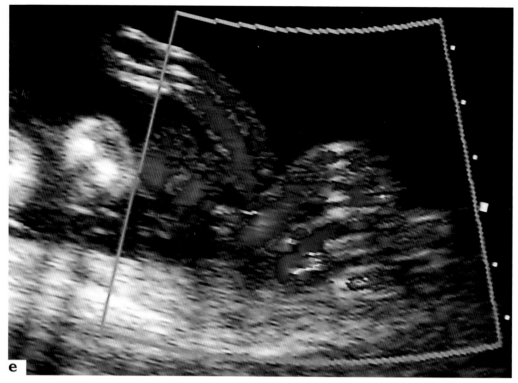

Figure 2.9 continued

(e) CDI shows that these entangled cords are velamentously inserted and that the twins had antepartum TTT. Note the differences in cord size (see also Figure 3.20 b)

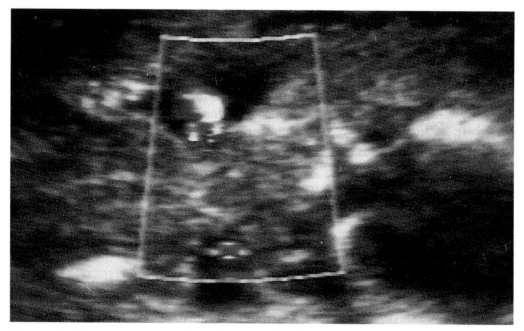

Figure 2.10 Intrapartum cord problems in MC, MA twins: One fetus has died *in utero*, but there is still pulsatile flow in a nuchal cord. Clearly, the cord is that of the surviving MC, MA co-twin

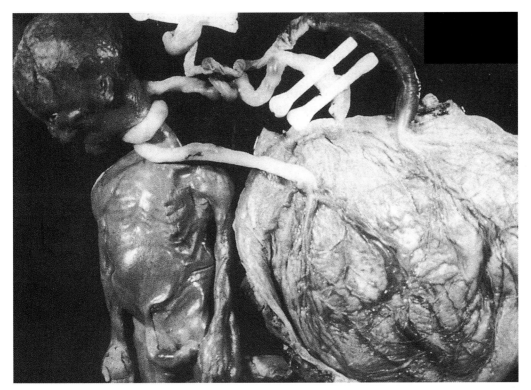

Figure 2.11 Intrapartum cord problems in MC, MA twins: Two loops of the living twin's cord are tightly wrapped around the neck of the dead fetus. In addition, the two cords were knotted. The surviving twin developed multiple sequelae of prematurity and asphyxia

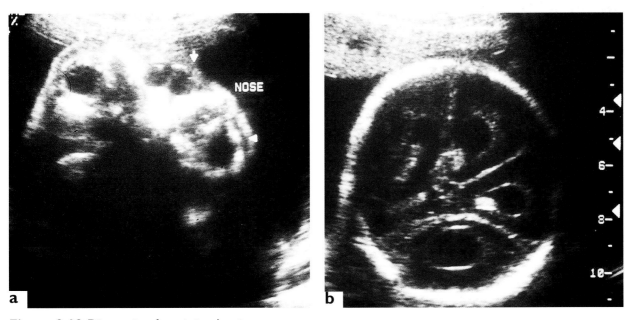

Figure 2.12 Diagnosis of conjoined twins:
(a) Ultrasonogram showing diprosopus twins (two faces in one head) with two noses, larger orbits lateral to each nose and smaller orbits between them;
(b) Ultrasonogram showing the complex brain structure of the twins

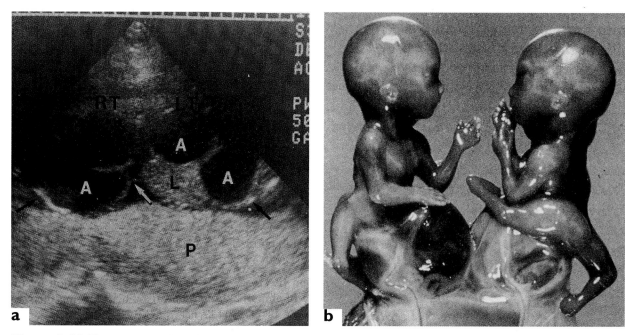

Figure 2.13 Twins concordant for congenital anomaly:
  (a) Ultrasonogram showing an anterior abdominal wall defect in each fetus;
  (b) Gross appearances show cloacal exstrophy in both twins

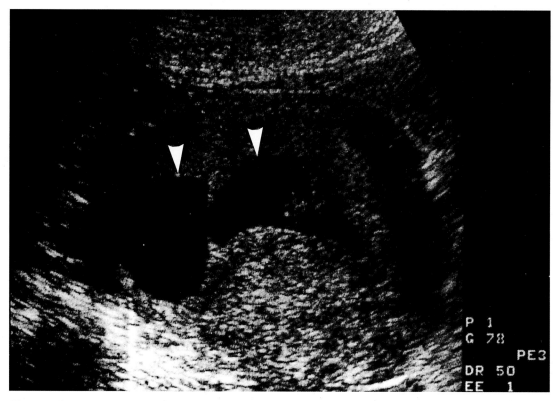

Figure 2.14 Antenatal diagnosis by chorionic villus sampling: In this ultrasonogram taken in the first trimester, the delta sign is well seen and both choria can be sampled (arrowed) by the transabdominal route

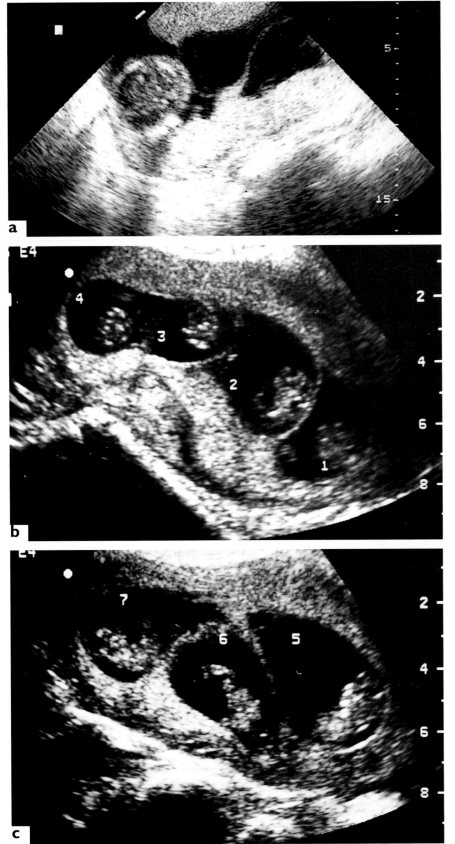

Figure 2.15 Antenatal diagnosis of higher-order multiple pregnancy (HOMP):

(a) Ultrasonogram of naturally conceived trichorionic (TC) MZ triplets shows the thick septa and two delta signs;

(b & c) Ultrasonograms of septachorionic septuplets as a result of ovulation induction. (It was not possible to visualize all seven sacs in one transducer plane.) In this case, the septuplets are septachorionic, but this does not exclude monozygosity of some of the pairs, as IVF and ovulation-induced HOMPs often contain MZ (including MC) twin pairs

Part I, Section 3 Understanding the pathology of twin pregnancies

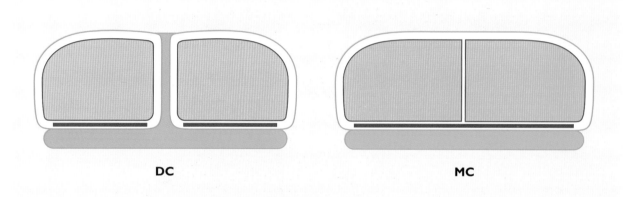

DC   MC

Figure 3.1 Fused DC contrasted with MC placentas: Fused DC (left) and MC (right) placentas. The septum of the DC placenta contains chorion (green), which prevents communication between the vessels (red) lying between the chorion and the amnion. In contrast, the septum of the MC placenta contains no chorion. Most MC placentas have various types of interfetal vascular anastomoses

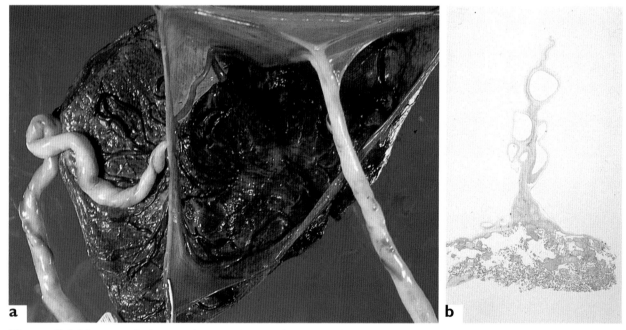

a   b

Figure 3.2 The septal chorion forms a barrier between the circulations of DC twins:

(a) In this fused DC placenta, both cords are inserted velamentously into the septum. Despite their close proximity, the vessels remain segregated by the septal chorion;

(b) Histology of the septum shows dilated fetal vessels running beneath the amnion on either side of the septal chorion, but remaining segregated. [Hematoxylin & eosin (H & E) stain]

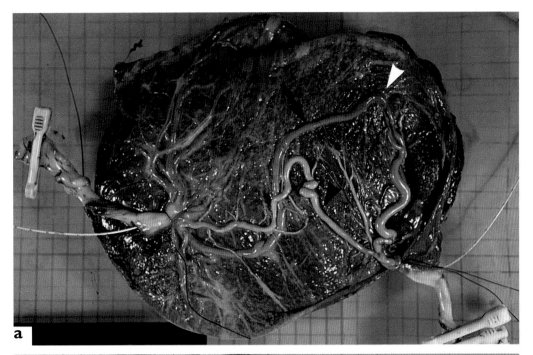

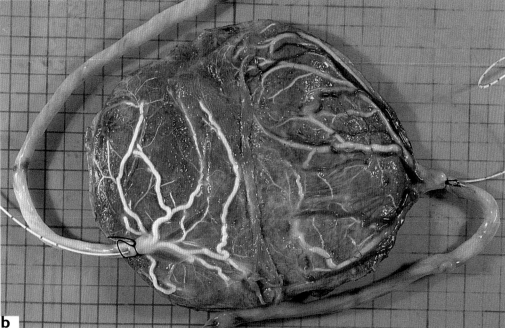

Figure 3.3 Patterns of vascular anastomoses and parenchymal sharing seen in typical injection studies of MC placentas:

(a) In this placenta, there is a large a↔a anastomosis (green; black arrow) and an a→v anastomosis (white arrow) between an artery of twin B (to the right) and a vein (dyed pink) of twin A. This combination of a↔a with a→v anastomosis is the most common pattern seen in MC placentas. Note the long course taken by the vein (pink; long arrow) back to the cord of twin A (to the left), indicating unequal venous sharing;

(b) Approximately 10% of MC placentas have no anastomoses. In this example, there is equal parenchymal sharing;

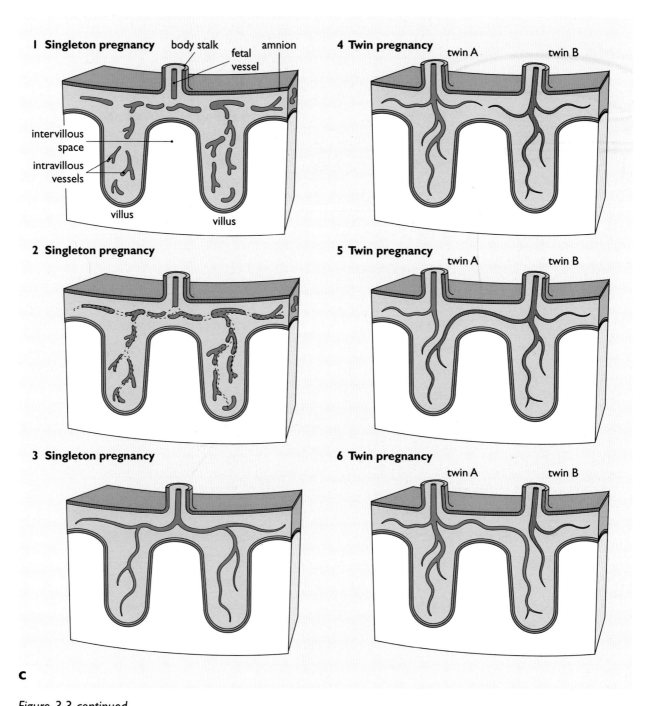

c

Figure 3.3 continued

(c) Independent development of the fetal and placental circulations, which later coalesce in the area of the body stalk (**1**); uncomplicated coalescence as seen in a singleton pregnancy (**2**&**3**); in contrast, with MC twin placentas the patterns of connections between the two fetal circulations and the common placental circulation are so variable that every MC twin placenta in fact has a unique pattern of vascularization (**4–6**). The pattern probably depends on the pattern of blood flow at the time the connections were made. Varying degrees of unequal vascular sharing may occur and are further complicated by anastomotic vessels (not shown here)

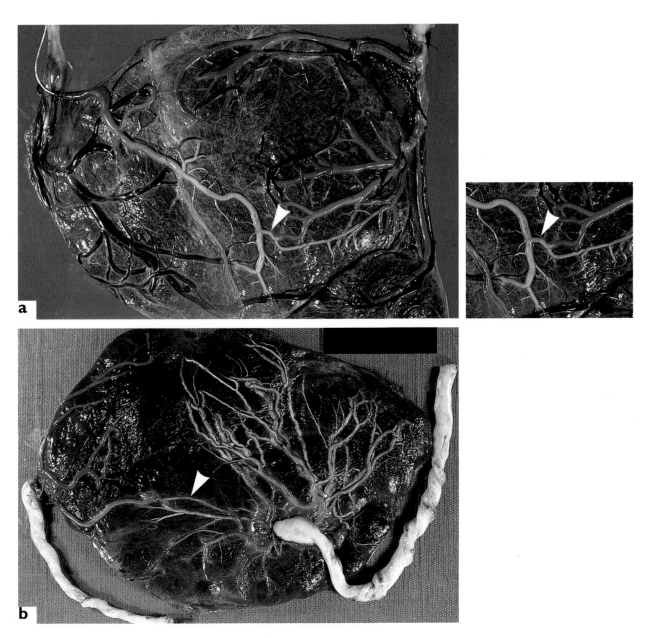

Figure 3.4 MC placentas with unequal vascular sharing:

(a) This placenta has a single a↔a anastomosis (yellow; arrow) between twin A (to the left) and twin B (to the right; see inset). The veins of twin A (dark blue) reach well beyond the point of the a↔a anastomosis towards twin B and drain parenchymal zones perfused by arteries of both twins. Thus, there are multiple sites of a→v anastomosis from twin B to twin A. The result in this case was growth discordance (of 26%; twins A and B weighed 2470 g and 1905 g, respectively) with unequal venous sharing in the presence of an a↔a anastomosis. There was no TTT. Both cords are velamentously inserted;

(b) This placenta shows markedly unequal venous sharing. Twin A (to the left) weighed 1980 g. Her arterial (pink) and venous (blue) zones were similar in size, and both covered a much smaller proportion of parenchyma than those of twin B (dyed yellow and green, respectively), who weighed 2560 g (23% growth discordance). There is an a↔a anastomosis (arrow), but no v↔v or a→v anastomotic zones. Therefore, there was no development of chronic antepartum TTT. The smaller parenchymal share of twin A may be correlated with the marginal cord insertion

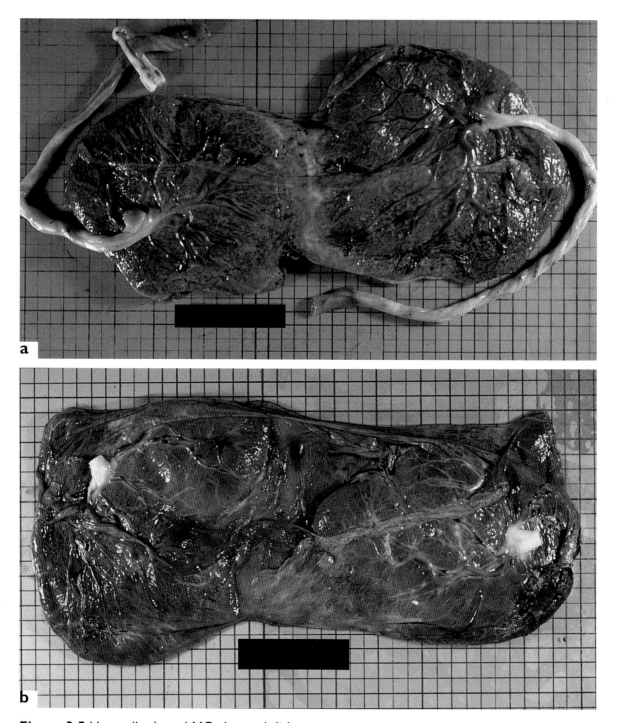

Figure 3.5 Unusually shaped MC placental disks:

(a) A narrow bridge of parenchymal tissue connects the two masses, and may cause an erroneous ultrasound diagnosis of fused DC placentas. This reinforces the dictum that the number of disks or partial disks does not necessarily correspond with chorion status (or zygosity);

(b) On rare occasions, MC disks are completely bilobar and connected by a membranous chorion which is unlikely to contain anastomoses. Such an MC placenta may be antenatally mistaken for DC placentas, albeit separate

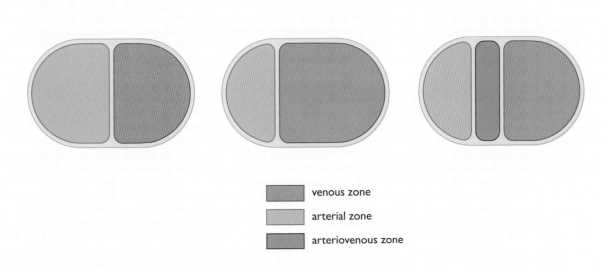

venous zone

arterial zone

arteriovenous zone

Figure 3.6 Schematic diagram of the vascular effects of unequal sharing of placental parenchyma:

(left) The size of the arterial (a) zone of twin A (blue) is equal to that of the venous (v) zone of twin B (red), and the venous zone of twin A is equal to that of the arterial zone of twin B. Thus, $a_A = v_A = a_B = v_B$ (see Figure 3.3 b); this is why growth discordance did not occur;

(middle) The arterial (a) and venous (v) zones of twin A (blue) are smaller than those of twin B (red). Thus, $a_A = v_A < a_B = v_B$ (see Figure 3.4). The result is nutritional growth discordance (A < B) which may or may not be modified by the presence or absence of anastomoses. In Figure 3.4, there were a ↔ a anastomoses and the twins were growth-discordant;

(right) The arterial (a) zone of twin A (blue) is larger than its venous (v) zone and the venous zone of twin B (red) is also larger than its arterial zone. Thus, $a_A > v_A$ and $a_B < v_B$. This paradox creates a *Grenzzone* or 'no-man's land' (purple) wherein a strip of parenchyma is supplied by arteries from twin A, but the blood is drained back into the veins of twin B. The clinical outcome of such an arrangement depends on the presence or absence of superficial anastomoses, as deep a → v anastomoses are, by definition, present. In Figure 3.4 a, an a ↔ a anastomosis is present, thus sparing the twins from uncompensated a → v transfusion and the development of chronic antenatal TTT. IN THE ABSENCE OF SUPERFICIAL ANASTOMOSES, HOWEVER, CHRONIC ANTENATAL TTT IS THE INEVITABLE CLINICAL RESULT OF THIS ARRANGEMENT (see Part I, Section 3, *Mechanisms of twin–twin transfusion*)

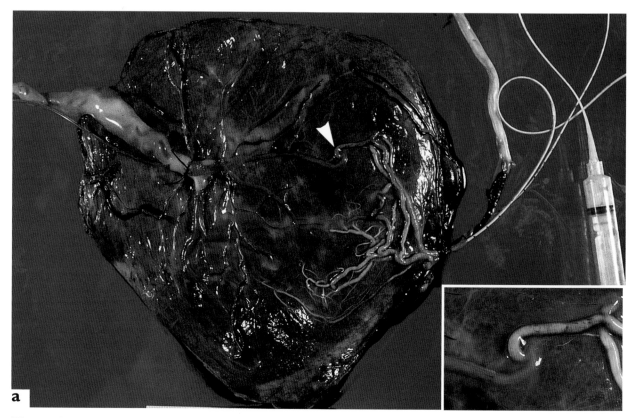

Figure 3.7 MC placental vascular anatomy in chronic antenatal TTT:

(a) Placenta of twins who died because of antenatal TTT complicated by acute reversed intrapartum TTT (see Figure 3.10b–f). The cord of the recipient, twin A (on the left), is central, large and congested whereas the cord of the donor, twin B (on the right), is velamentous, thin and pale. Venous sharing is unequal, with the venous zone of twin A (pink) radiating from the central cord and greatly exceeding that of donor twin B (green). No superficial (a↔a or v↔v) anastomoses are seen, but there is a single a→v anastomosis (arrow) between an artery of twin B (orange) and a vein of twin A (pink; see inset). This anastomosis is in an area where the larger venous perfusion zone of the recipient twin overlaps the arterial perfusion of the donor twin; (inset) The anastomosing vessels meet 'nose-to-nose', but no transfer of dye occurs in the large vessels at the surface. The anastomosis is deep within the parenchyma of a cotyledon;

(b) In another case of TTT, a single a→v anastomosis (arrow) connects the donor (left) and recipient (right). Parenchymal congestion is seen on the side of the recipient;

(c) Parenchymal congestion is clearly visible on the maternal surface;

(d) Anatomy of a→v anastomoses: The cord of the left twin is centrally inserted and that of the right twin is marginal/velamentous (usually corresponding to the donor). **1** shows two pairs of arteries and veins, one from each twin, approaching the placental equator before penetrating the chorionic plate to enter the parenchyma. Each artery/vein pair does this through a single foramen. There is no anastomosis. This is the usual vascular pattern to cotyledons of all placentas, whether singleton or twin. **2** shows a simple, superficial, a↔a anastomosis. The arteries are usually not accompanied by corresponding veins. **3** shows a simple, superficial, v↔v anastomosis, the veins unaccompanied by corresponding arteries; **4** and **5** show bidirectional a→v anastomoses. In each case, the contributing artery and vein are not accompanied by a corresponding vein and artery of that twin. The artery and vein inappropriately penetrate the chorionic plate close together (nose-to-nose; see a above) in a pattern similar to that seen in appropriate arteries and veins of the same twin. The vessels do not join on the surface. Functional anastomosis takes place at the level of the villous vessels in the parenchyma;

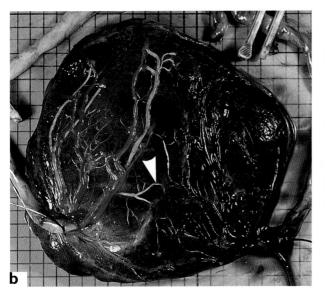

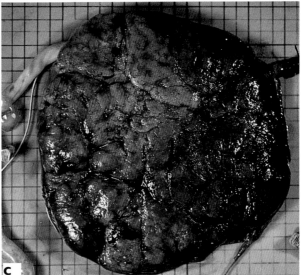

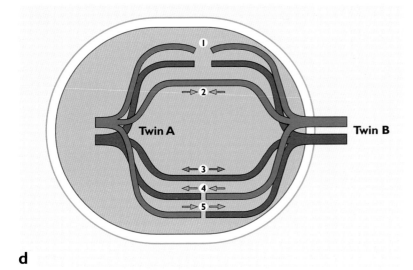

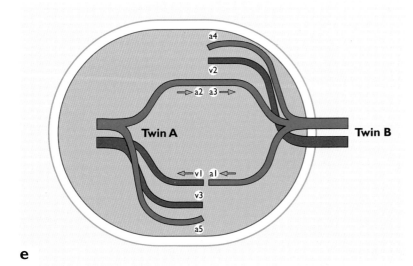

(e) This shows the most common anastomotic combination: a → v with a ↔ a. Both twins independently perfuse separate zones of the placenta, via v3 and a5 of twin A, and a4 and v2 of twin B. In addition, there is a unidirectional a → v anastomosis from twin B to twin A, via one arterial branch of twin B (a1) and one venous branch of twin A (v1). The return a ↔ a anastomosis (from a2 of twin A to a3 of twin B) protects the twins from the effects of the a → v anastomosis, but not without cost. The net result of the four vessels of twin A is two zones of venous return, v1 and v3, for the production of two arterial zones, a2 and a5. For twin B, however, the four vessels comprise two normal arterial outputs, but only one venous return. This twin also receives arterial blood from twin A via the a ↔ a anastomosis, but this blood is relatively deoxygenated and depleted of nutrients. Apart from the fact that the donor of the a → v anastomosis frequently has a marginal/velamentous cord insertion (as shown here), the donor may experience further growth discordance because of this anastomotic imbalance

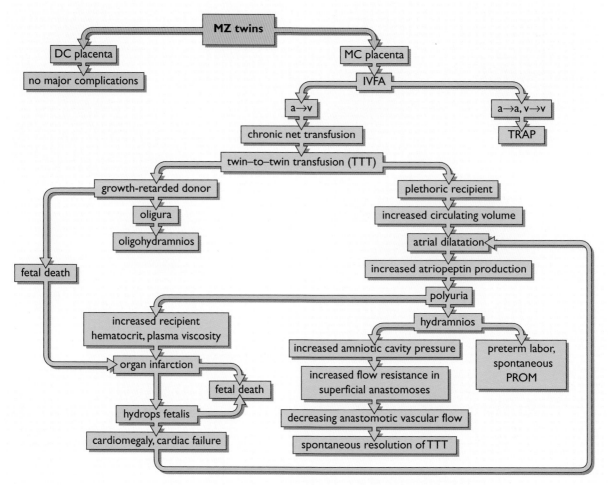

a

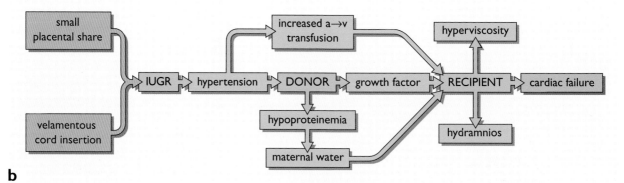

b

Figure 3.8 Cascade of events leading to severe antepartum TTT, its consequences and new modes of treatment:

(a) After the initial transfusion, several events follow in the donor and recipient. Some are transmitted from donor to recipient via placental anastomoses;

(b) Other events involve maternal water and electrolytes. The results are the oligohydramniotic, 'stuck', undergrown donor twin and the plethoric/hydropic and hydramniotic recipient. Biophysical deterioration of either twin is likely to affect the co-twin as well

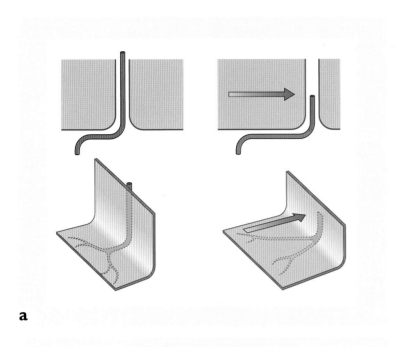

a

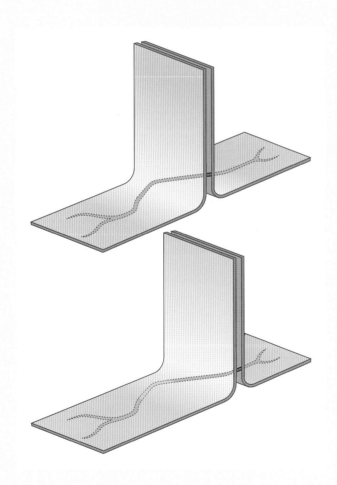

b

Figure 3.9 Effects of hydramnios and therapeutic amniocentesis in antepartum TTT:

(a) Onset of hydramnios expands the sac of the recipient and shifts the septum in relation to the chorionic plate, shown diagrammatically in (upper) lateral and (lower) superolateral oblique views. At the same time, vessels (particularly veins) running velamentously in the septum may be stretched and occluded;

(b) With normally inserted cords, shifting of the septum may allow the transmission of pressure to a patent v↔v connection (pink; upper) with occlusion (blue segment; lower) of this possible route of compensation for an a→v transfusion;

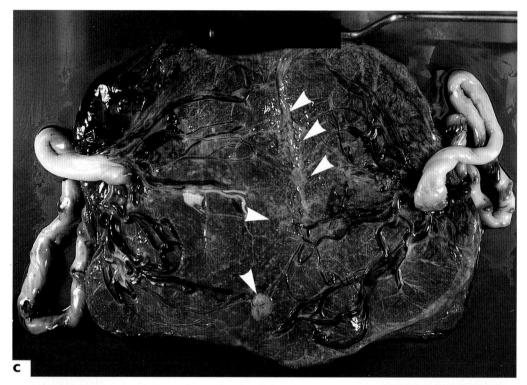

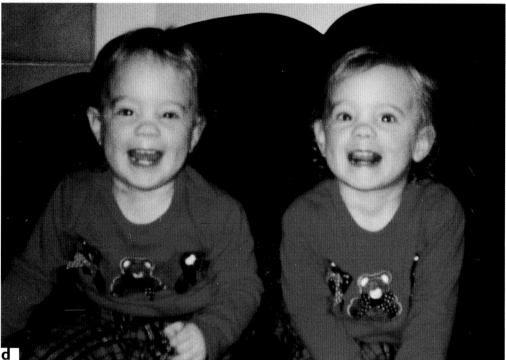

Figure 3.9 continued
(c) Appearance of placenta after laser occlusion of vessels for treatment of chronic antepartum TTT. The coagulation zones (arrows) are distributed across the equator and have effectively segregated the two fetal circulations;
(d) At age 36 months, the twins show no evidence of sequelae of TTT

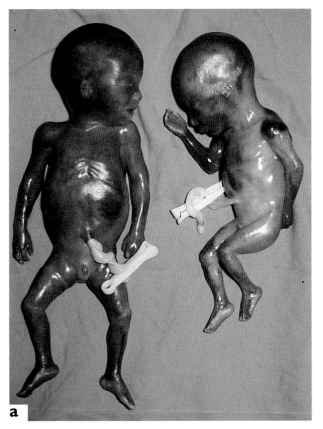

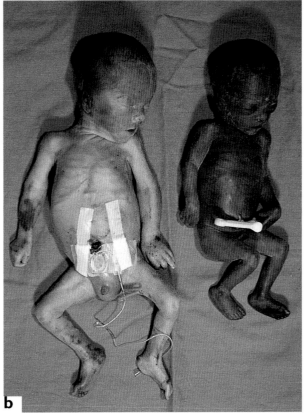

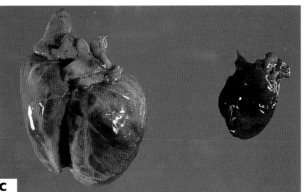

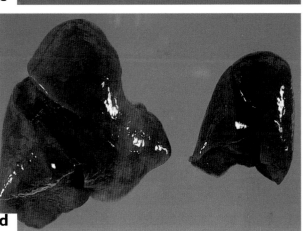

Figure 3.10 Effects of antepartum TTT on twins and their organs:

(a) Double fetal death due to antepartum TTT. The recipient (left) is large and plethoric with limbs and trunk in extension, indicative of hydramnios. The donor (right) is smaller, pale and fixed in flexion, the result of being 'stuck' secondary to oligo-hydramnios.

(b) Twins showing the appropriate growth discordance seen with antepartum TTT. There was also superimposed acute peripartum TTT following cord-clamping of the first-born larger twin (left), with the chronic donor twin (right) appearing paradoxically plethoric. This was because of acute drainage of blood from the MC placenta into twin B in the interval between clamping of the cords. There were large differences in organ sizes and weights;

(c) Circulatory overload from hypervolemia and hyperviscosity caused right ventricular hypertrophy in the chronic recipient (left). In survivors, such hypertrophy may either slowly regress or prove fatal;

(d) Similar size discordance is seen in the lungs;

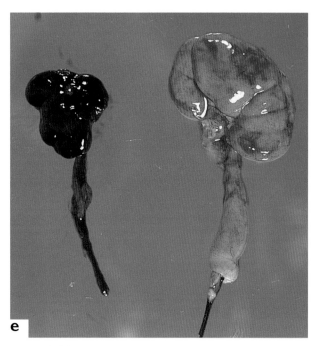
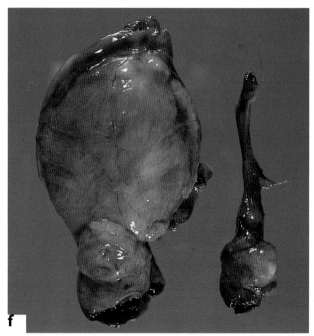

Figure 3.10 continued

(e) Kidneys are particularly discordant because of the oliguria and polyuria affecting the chronic donor (left) and recipient (right), respectively;

(f) Polyuria and oliguria are also reflected in the respective bladder sizes of the chronic recipient (left) and donor (right)

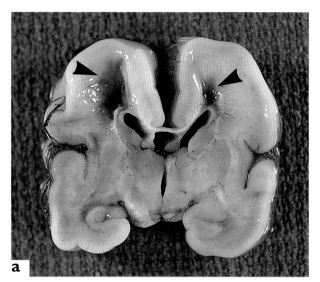
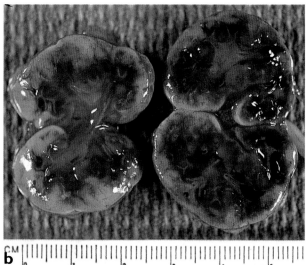

Figure 3.11 Effects of fetal death of one MC twin on the surviving twin: There was TTT with hydramnios/oligohydramnios and growth discordance. The smaller twin died 10 days before delivery of the co-twin, who developed oliguria/oligohydramnios in the interim. The survivor lived for only a few minutes;

(a) The longer-lived twin had bilateral cavitating periventriclar leukomalacia, as seen in this coronal brain section, and

(b) Bilateral renal necrosis;

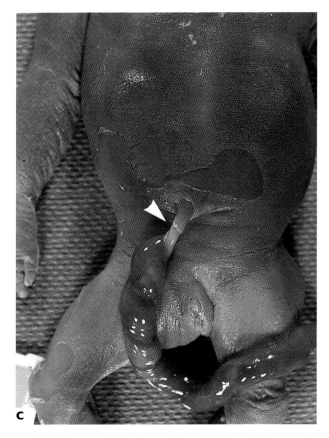

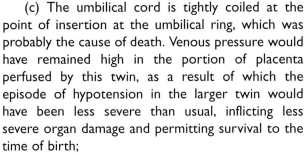

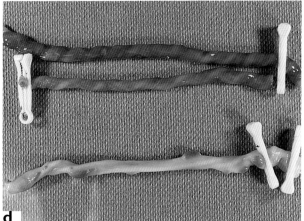

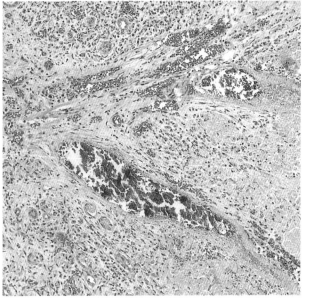

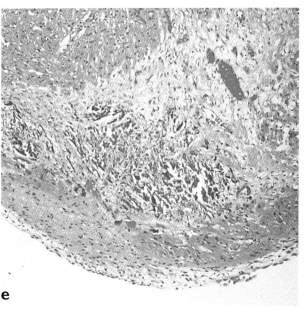

(c) The umbilical cord is tightly coiled at the point of insertion at the umbilical ring, which was probably the cause of death. Venous pressure would have remained high in the portion of placenta perfused by this twin, as a result of which the episode of hypotension in the larger twin would have been less severe than usual, inflicting less severe organ damage and permitting survival to the time of birth;

(d) Comparison of the cords of the twins;

(e) Histology (H & Es) of the kidney (upper) shows bland infarction and calcification of the walls of the arcuate arteries, suggesting a previous thrombotic episode. Histology of the heart (lower), which was massively enlarged by right ventricular hypertrophy, shows multifocal ischemic necrosis and scarring with dystrophic calcification. These ischemic lesions almost certainly date from the time of death of the co-twin 10 days previously. However, it is unusual for the smaller twin to die first and the co-twin, if affected by an episode of hypotension and organ ischemia, usually dies soon after. In this case, the death of the smaller twin may not have been directly due to TTT

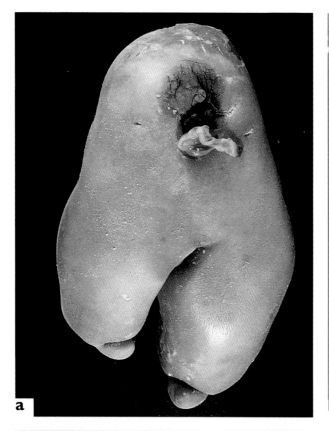

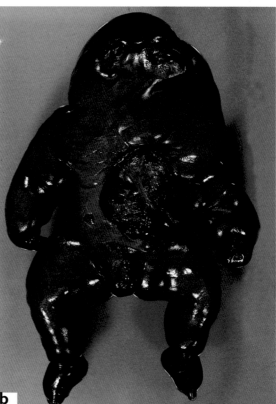

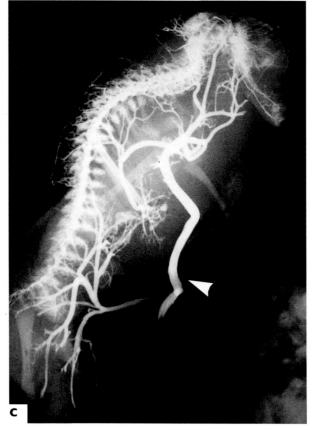

Figure 3.12 Holoacardius acephalus:

(a) Typical appearances of an acardius acephalus fetus with absence of a head and arms;

(b) Acardiac fetuses are often hydropic. Dissection of the internal organs demonstrates a simplified alimentary tract whereas the thoracic viscera are absent or vestigial;

(c) Retrograde umbilical arteriography shows a large abnormal (?vitelline) artery (arrow) entering the trunk and apparently branching into primitive branchial arch arteries. There is no evidence of a heart or dorsal aorta

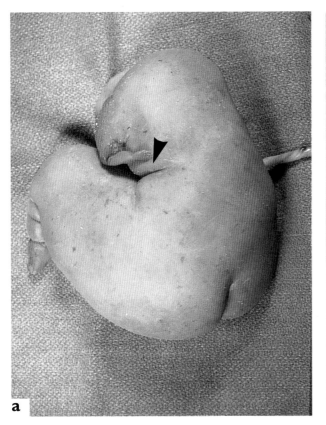

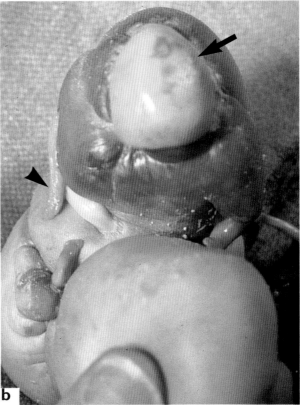

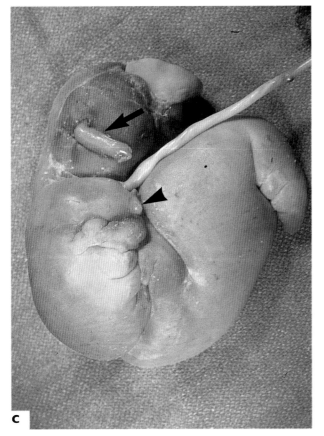

Figure 3.13 Acardiac fetuses may show regression of body parts:

(a) Left lateral view of an apparently simplified torso and legs; note the reduced left arm (arrow);

(b) Frontal view shows the brain (long arrow) to be an area of liquified yellow tissue. The right arm (arrow) shows evidence of 'mummification', as does the right foot [see (c)];

(c) Right lateral view shows the brain, right arm (long arrow) and right foot (arrow). The left leg is not reduced. These appearances suggest that early brain and limb development was normal. However, a sudden hemodynamic event resulted in rapid peripheral vascular shut-down, and symmetrical hypoperfusion of the brain and distal extremities

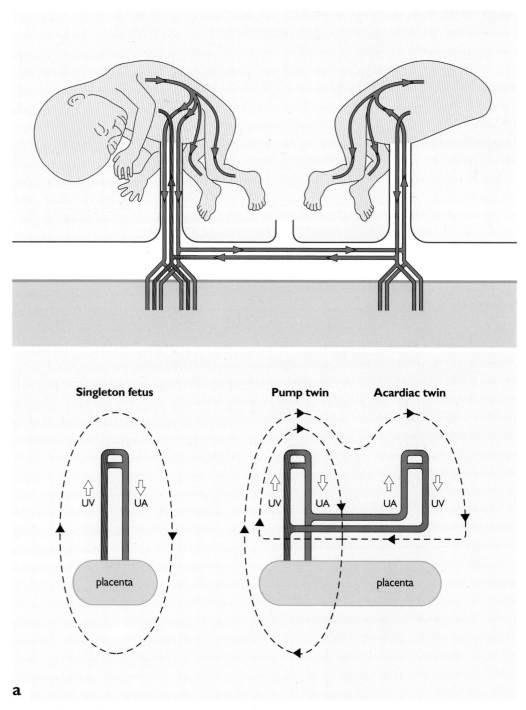

a

Figure 3.14 Placental vasculature in acardiac and 'pump' twins:

(a) Schematic diagram of transplacental vascular relationships of a pump twin and its co-twin, the acardiac fetus. Umbilical arterial blood (blue) from the pump twin, crossing via an a↔a anastomosis above the chorionic plate (green) and beneath the amnion (pink), flows in a retrograde direction up the umbilical artery of the acardiac twin and usually reaches the aorta via common iliac or vitelline arteries. Blood (purple) returning to the pump twin via the v↔v anastomosis has been doubly perfused through the bodies of both twins without passing through the placenta;

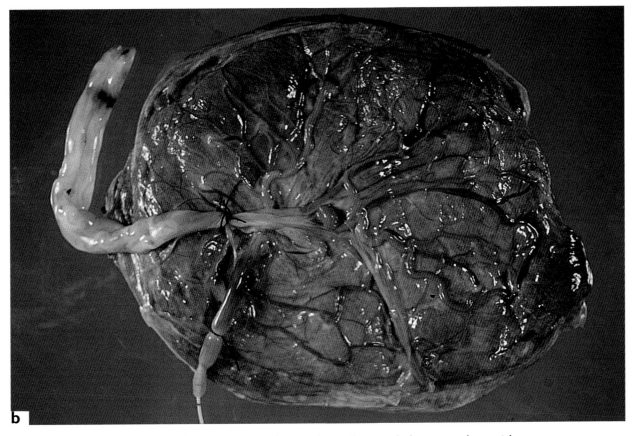

(b) In the placenta in acardiac pregnancy, the cords are inserted close together, with large a↔a (dyed pink) and v↔v (dyed blue) anastomoses. These are the necessary vascular anatomical conditions for development and maintenance of TRAP

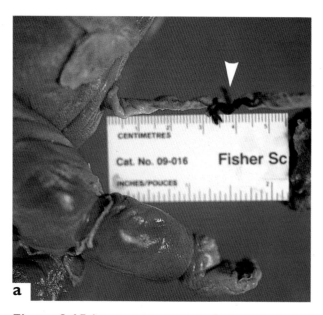

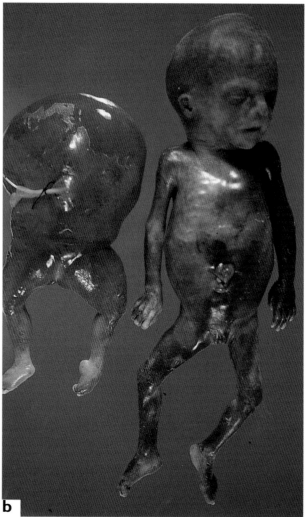

Figure 3.15 Intrauterine surgery for acardiac twin pregnancy:

(a) The cord of this acardiac fetus was ligated (arrow) *in utero* at 24 weeks of gestation. Labor ensued 10 days later, and the pump twin survived albeit with complications of prematurity;

(b) In another case, the cord of the acardiac fetus was successfully occluded with a Filshie clip in the antenatal period. However, early labor unresponsive to tocolytic therapy soon followed, and the pump twin succumbed to the preterm delivery (same fetus as in Figures 3.12c and 3.14b)

Figure 3.16 (*facing page*) Correlation between MC placental vascular anatomy and clinical outcome: Outcomes are strongly related to patterns of vascular anastomoses and vascular sharing. Data obtained from a series of 69 MC twin pregnancies show:

(a) When vessels were assessed for the presence/absence of various types of anastomoses and for equal/unequal venous sharing, the resultant 13 vascular arrangements were found with the frequencies shown here;

(b) Perinatal mortality (%) with each vascular pattern. The presence of a→v anastomosis without compensatory superficial a↔a or v↔v anastomosis was the cause of antepartum TTT, resulting in high mortality;

TYPES	No a↔a or v↔v present	a↔a present	v↔v present	a↔a and v↔v present
Equal venous, no a→v present	1 — 13 (19%)	2 — 2 (3%)		3 — 3 (4%)
Unequal venous, arterial corresponding, no a→v present	4 — 3 (4%)	5 — 2 (3%)		6 — 2 (3%)
Equal venous, a→v present, unidirectional	7 — 8 (12%)	8 — 6 (9%)	9 — 1 (1%)	10 — 1 (1%)
Unequal venous, arterial non-corresponding, a→v present, bidirectional	11 — 2 (3%)			
Unequal venous, arterial non-corresponding, a→v present, unidirectional	12 — 6 (9%)	13 — 17 (25%)	14 — 1 (1%)	15 — 2 (3%)

a

PERINATAL MORTALITY	No a↔a or v↔v present	a↔a present	v↔v present	a↔a and v↔v present
Equal venous, no a→v present	1 — 7.7%	2 — 0%		3 — 0%
Unequal venous, arterial corresponding, no a→v present	4 — 16%	5 — 0%		6 — 0%
Equal venous, a→v present, unidirectional	7 — 25%	8 — 0%	9 — 0%	10 — 0%
Unequal venous, arterial non-corresponding, a→v present, bidirectional	11 — 50%			
Unequal venous, arterial non-corresponding, a→v present, unidirectional	12 — 83%	13 — 9%	14 — 0%	15 — 0%

b

HYDRAMNIOS	No a↔a or v↔v present	a↔a present	v↔v present	a↔a and v↔v present
Equal venous, no a→v present	1 0%	2 0%		3 0%
Unequal venous, arterial corresponding, no a→v present	4 0%	5 25%		6 0%
Equal venous, a→v present, unidirectional	7 25%	8 0%	9 100%	10 0%
Unequal venous, arterial non–corresponding, a→v present, bidirectional	11 0%			
Unequal venous, arterial non-corresponding, a→v present, unidirectional	12 100%	13 12%	14 100%	15 50%

c

GESTATIONAL AGE	No a↔a or v↔v present	a↔a present	v↔v present	a↔a and v↔v present
Equal venous, no a→v present	1 34.3	2 34.0		3 35.7
Unequal venous, arterial corresponding, no a→v present	4 34.7	5 35.5		6 33.0
Equal venous, a→v present, unidirectional	7 32.0	8 35.0	9 29.0	10 37.0
Unequal venous, arterial non–corresponding, a→v present, bidirectional	11 34.5			
Unequal venous, arterial non-corresponding, a→v present, unidirectional	12 26.7	13 34.9	14 33.0	15 33.5

d

Figure 3.16 continued
(c) Percentage of cases with hydramnios analyzed by vascular anatomy;
(d) Mean gestational age (weeks) with each type of vascular pattern;

GROWTH DISCORDANCE	No a↔a or v↔v present	a↔a present	v↔v present	a↔a and v↔v present
Equal venous, no a→v present	1 13%	2 8%		3 13%
Unequal venous, arterial corresponding, no a→v present	4 38%	5 47%		6 19%
Equal venous, a→v present, unidirectional	7 8%	8 5%	9 21%	10 15%
Unequal venous, arterial non–corresponding, a→v present, bidirectional	11 14%			
Unequal venous, arterial non-corresponding, a→v present, unidirectional	12 35%	13 13%	14 40%	15 37%

e

(e) Mean percentage growth discordance with each type of vascular pattern. In all analyses, isolated a→v anastomosis with unequal venous sharing caused the most mortality and morbidity

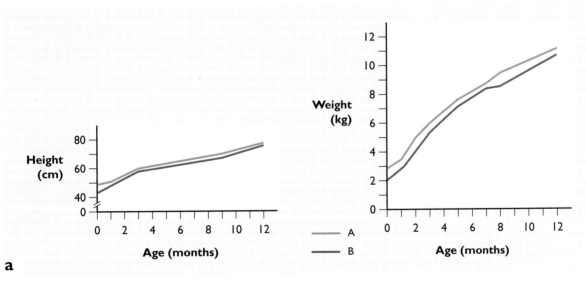

a

Figure 3.17 Growth discordance without TTT: These MC twins were growth discordant in mid-trimester, but had no evidence of chronic antepartum TTT. A diagnosis of unequal venous sharing was made, and response to the mother's strict bedrest was good. Delivery was at 36 weeks, when twin A weighed 2660 g and twin B weighed 1920 g (28% growth discordance);

(a) Body weight and length of the twins ran closely parallel for the first year of life without catch-up;

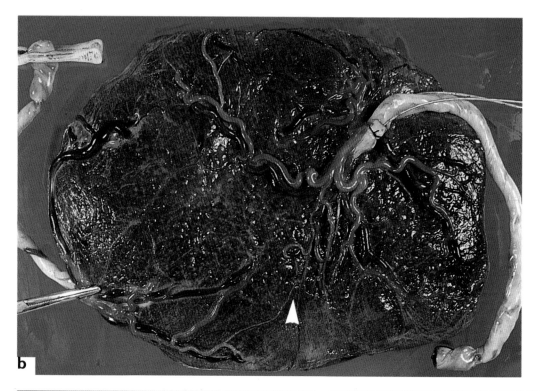

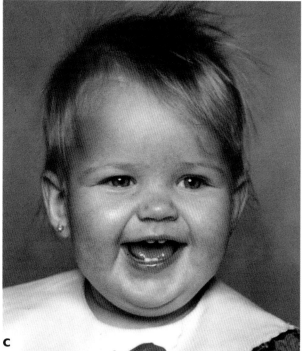

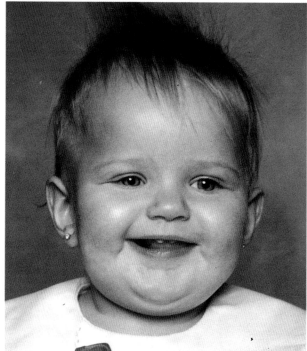

Figure 3.17 continued

(b) Placental injection confirms unequal venous sharing with one small a↔a anastomosis (arrow) and one area of potential a→v transfusion. The smaller twin (left) has a marginal cord insertion and a smaller share of the placental parenchyma;

(c) The twins at age 1 year. The larger twin (right), who was heavier at birth, continues the mesomorphic trend, with a fatter face and heavier build

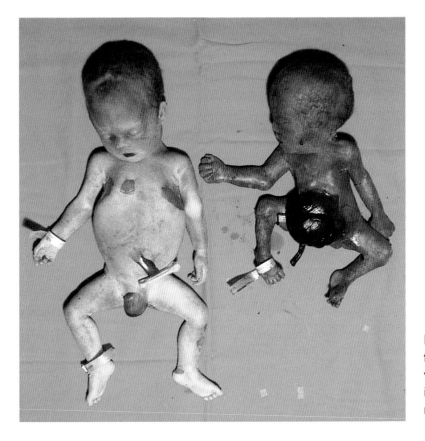

Figure 3.18 MC twins discordant for omphalocele. In addition, there was acute intrapartum TTT, resulting in the plethoric appearance of the malformed infant

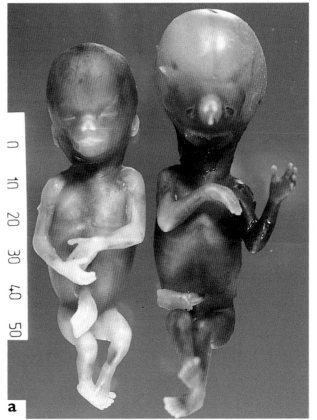

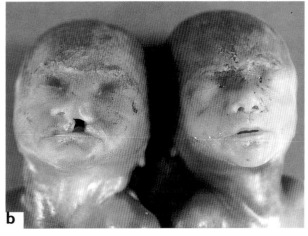

Figure 3.19 MC twins discordant for facial malformation:

(a) After spontaneous miscarrige at 14 weeks, the twin on the right shows holoprosencephaly/synotia whereas the co-twin is normal. TTT was present and the malformed fetus was the recipient;

(b) In another case, the malformed twin has a cleft lip and palate. Spontaneous delivery was at 23 weeks with chronic antenatal TTT

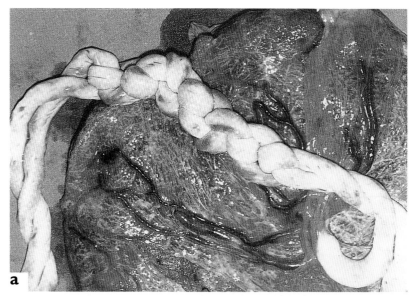

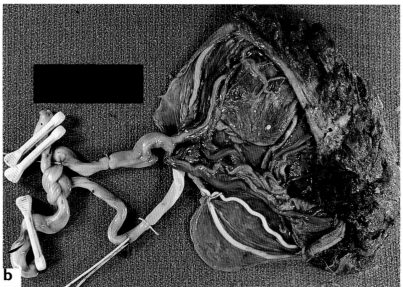

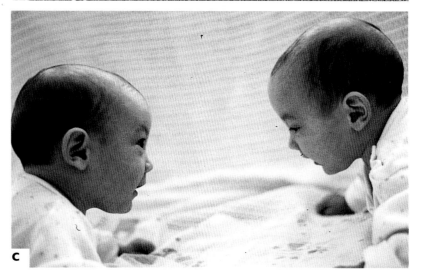

Figure 3.20 Risks in mono-amniotic (MA) twins:

(a) Complex braiding of cords occurs only in MA twins. In this case, both twins survived;

(b) In this MA placental disk in prenatal TTT, the cords were inserted velamentously, side-by-side, with complex braiding and knotting. The donor survived, but the recipient had right ventricular cardiomyopathy (see also Figure 2.9 e);

(c) These MA twins survived intact and had similar birth weights

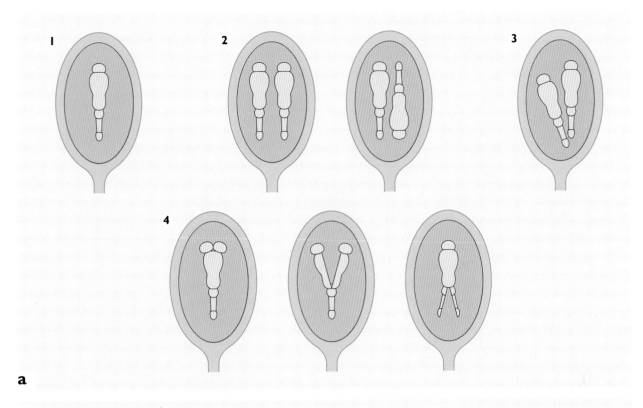

a

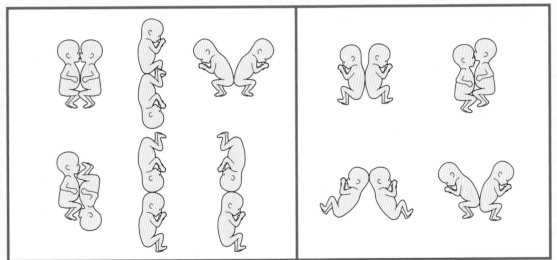

b

Figure 3.21 Schematic diagrams showing various arrangements of MC, MA and conjoined twins (CT), and their axes on the embryonic disk:

(a) **1** is a dorsal view of a singleton embryo; **2** shows twin MC, MA embryos with axes in parallel, either head-to-head or head-to-tail; **3** shows two embryos lying obliquely; **4** shows the classical axial arrangements considered to result in CT;

(b) Permitted types of CT (left) have notochords as far apart as possible, lying either ventroventrally, caudocaudally or craniocranially. The CT are segmentally 'in register'. In non-permitted types of CT (right), there is dorsodorsal notochordal incursion or lack of segmental registration;

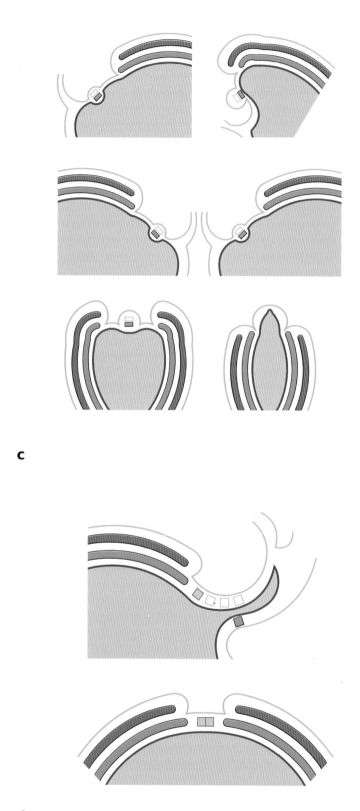

c

d

Figure 3.21 continued

(c) The cardiogenic zone and future septum transversum lie cranial to the cranial extent of the notochord and neural tube with the buccopharyngeal membrane intervening (upper). These parts travel ventrally and caudally during the formation of the headfold. When the fields of embryonic CT coalesce cranio-cranially (middle), the extent of overlap determines the type of CT. When coalescence is in the region of the cardiogenic zone and future septum transversum (lower left), there will be variable sharing of hearts and livers, making it difficult to surgically separate the thoracopagus CT. When coalescence is at the level of the buccopharyngal membrane (lower right), the hearts and livers are reconstituted laterally, using elements of both axes, rather than remaining ventral. The embryos will share a common Rathke's pouch and pharynx, as seen in cephalothoracopagus (janiceps) CT;

(d) Similar considerations apply to ischiopagus CT. Depending on the degree of overlap of the components of the cloacal membrane (anal, genital and urinary), some organs are reconstituted laterally rather than ventrally. Typically, a common anus is present, but genital and urinary tracts will empty laterally at the perineums, and the organs are formed from contributions of both axes;

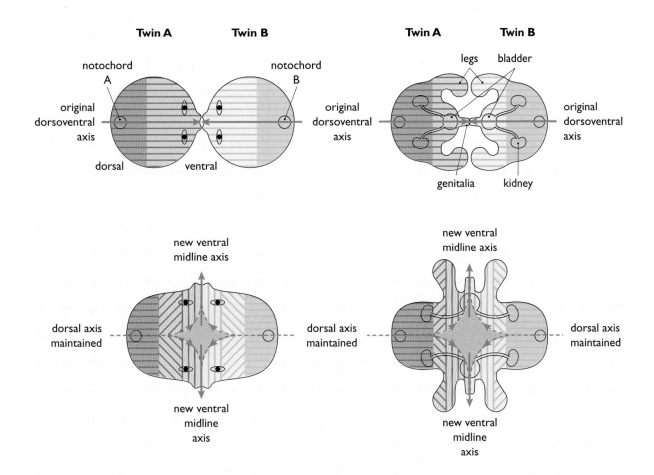

e

(e) In janiceps twins (left), the two notochordal axes are most closely apposed at the cranial end and steadily diverge caudally. At the cranial pole, there is minimal expression of the usual ventral organs, which are thrust laterally outwards to form new midline axes from components of each axis (biclonal). Proceeding downwards towards the caudal end, there are zones which now have sufficient space for ventral organs to form independently for each axis.

Similar considerations apply when there is close apposition of the two axes at the caudal end, as seen in ischiopagus twins (right). Caudally, new biclonal organs are constituted laterally outwards. There is a stronger tendency back towards the normal axial orientations on proceeding cranially;

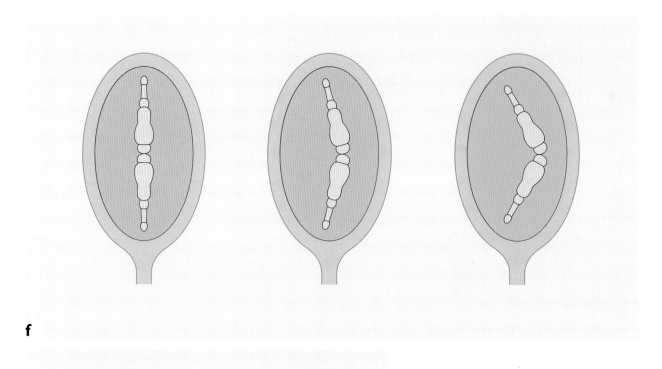

f

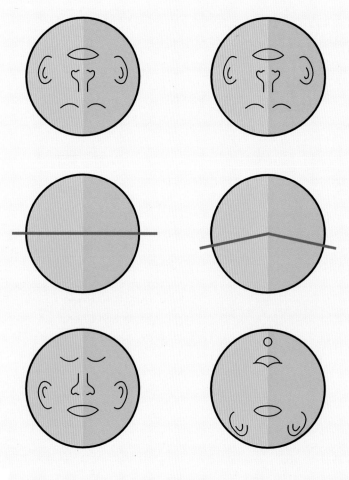

g

Figure 3.21 continued
(f) A further consideration is that the dorsoventral planes of the two CT axes are not always perfectly aligned at 180° on the embryonic disk; they may be non-congruent. In such cases, there is usually hypoplasia on the lesser side (cyclopia of the eye in janiceps or symmelia of the lower limbs in ischiopagus CT);

(g) Congruent (left) and non-congruent (right) axes in janiceps CT result in two fully developed biclonal faces (left), and a normal and a hypoplastic cyclopic face (right), respectively;

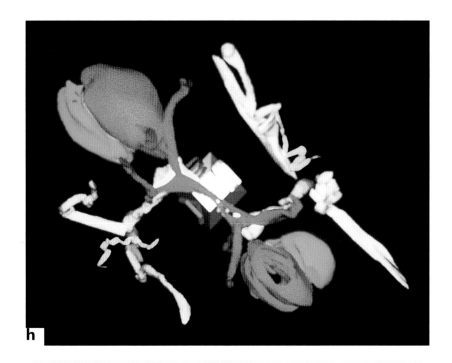

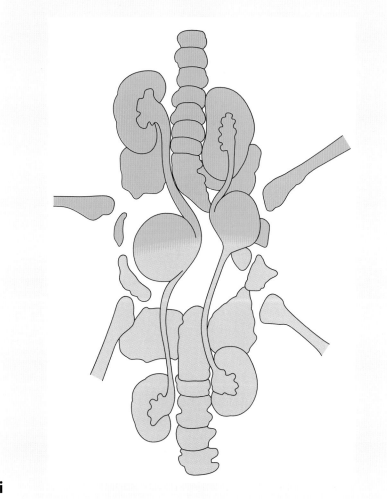

(h) Three-dimensional computer reconstruction of the organs in congruent janiceps CT. The notochords are yellow. The two hearts are orientated laterally in new axes, and there is an arterial anastomosis connecting the two aortic arches;

(i) Image taken from a pyelogram of ischiopagus CT shows the skeletons lying in two axes (pink and green). Each bladder receives the ureter of a kidney in each axis;

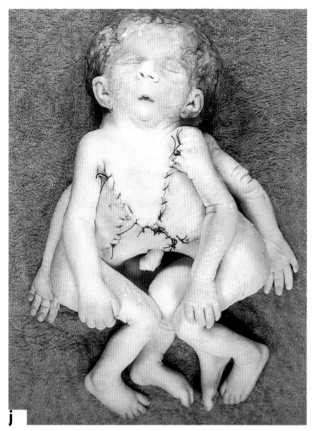

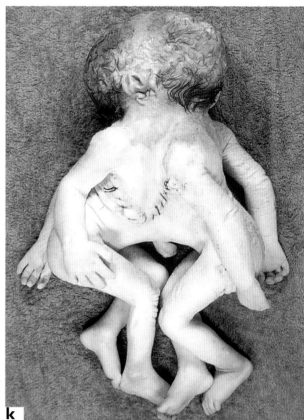

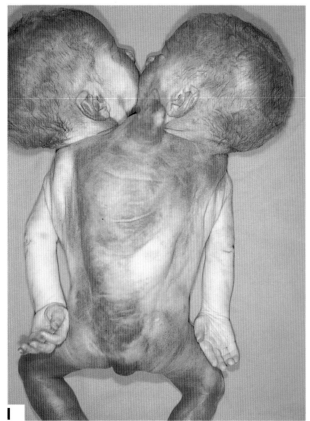

Figure 3.21 continued

(j) Non-congruent janiceps twins showing the complete face (non-hypoplastic side);

(k) On the opposite (hypoplastic) side, there are only two ears and no true facial components;

(l) Non-separable dicephalus CT

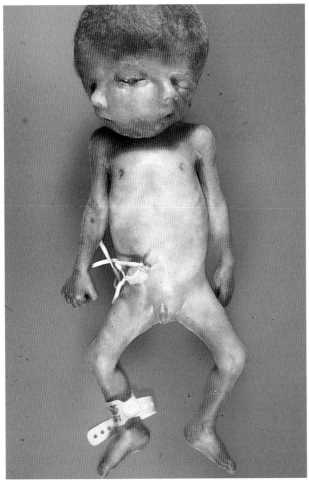

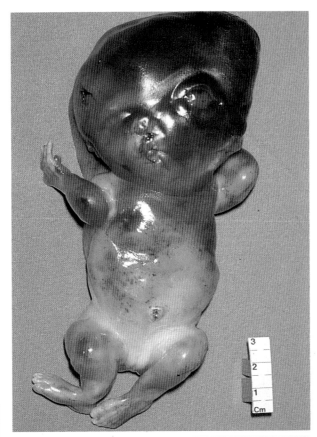

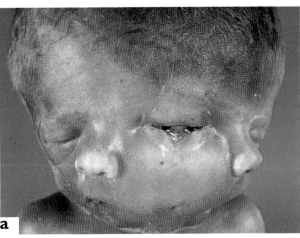

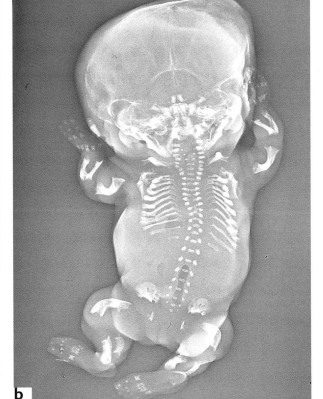

Figure 3.22 Examples of conjoined twins (CT):

(a) Diprosopus CT are the result of two noto-chordal axes lying closely parallel and side-by-side. There are two faces on one head (close-up, lower);

(b) Diprosopus CT with thanatophoric dwarfism (upper). Radiography (lower) shows features of type I thanatophoric dwarfism;

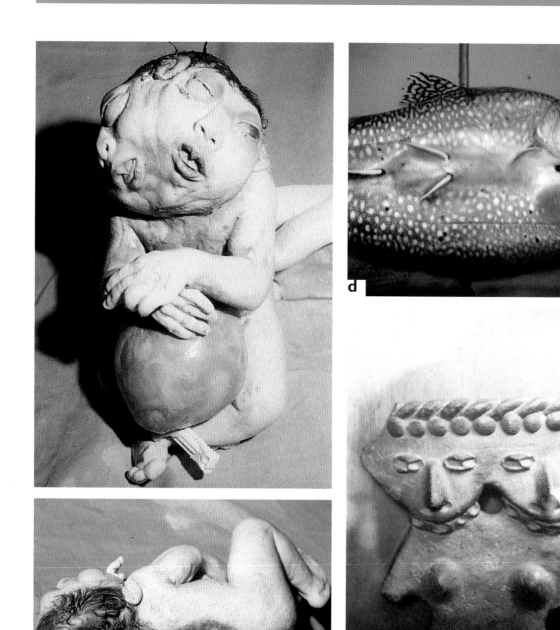

Figure 3.22 continued

(c) Diprosopus CT with omphalocele (upper) and extensive neural tube defect (lower; same fetus). These two midline malformations are examples of interaction aplasia wherein conflicting developmental 'instructions' from the two axes result in failure to complete body wall closure;

(d) A pair of thoracopagus trout;

(e) Dicephalic CT depicted in a neolithic terracotta figurine

Part II, Section I How to examine twin and HOMP placentas

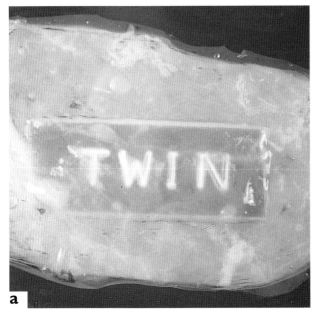
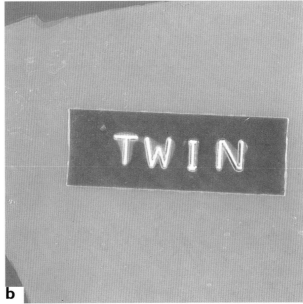
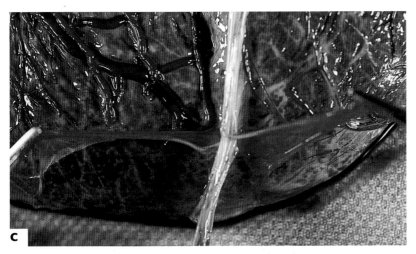
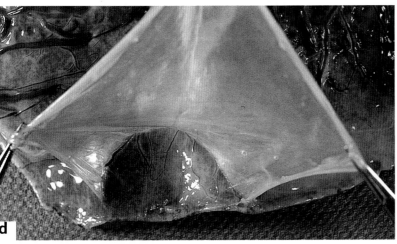

Figure 4.1 DC contrasted with MC septa:

(a) A DC septum (laid over a marker) is translucent, although yellow-orange fragments of chorionic villi can be seen;

(b) An MC septum is completely transparent;

(c) When the layers of a fused DC, DA placenta are teased apart at one end of the septum and the two amniotic layers peeled to either side, the central chorionic component remains firmly attached to the placental disk. The remainder of the septum is left intact for microscopic confirmation;

(d) With an MC, DA placenta, separation of the two amniotic layers leaves no other structure as the septum contains no chorionic component. These simple tests can be carried out in the delivery room

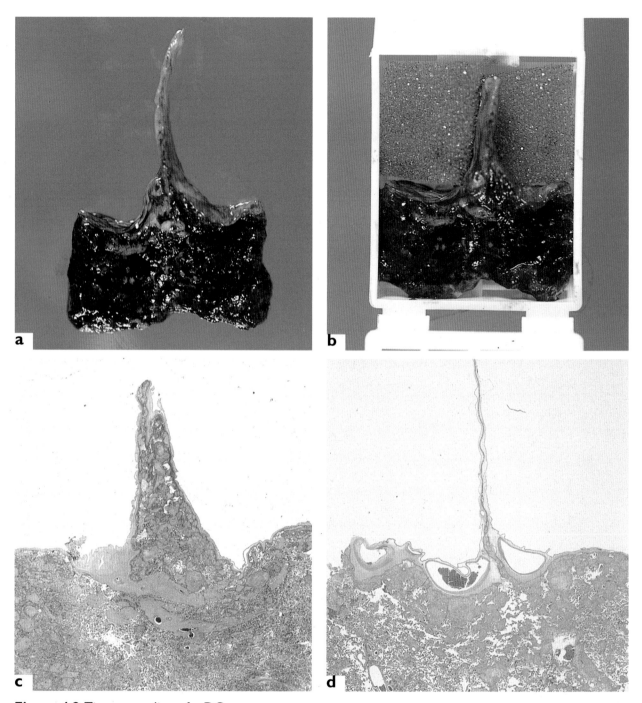

Figure 4.2 Tissue sampling of a DC septum:

(a) A slice of membranous septum is cut at the T-junction. The region corresponding to the delta sign is clearly seen;

(b) When embedding the specimen, the section is carefully laid in the cassette, ensuring that the septum is at right angles to the placental surface;

(c) The corresponding tissue section (H&E) shows a prominent delta sign and a thick septum;

(d) In a tissue section from another case (H&E), the septum is thinner, but the delta sign is still evident

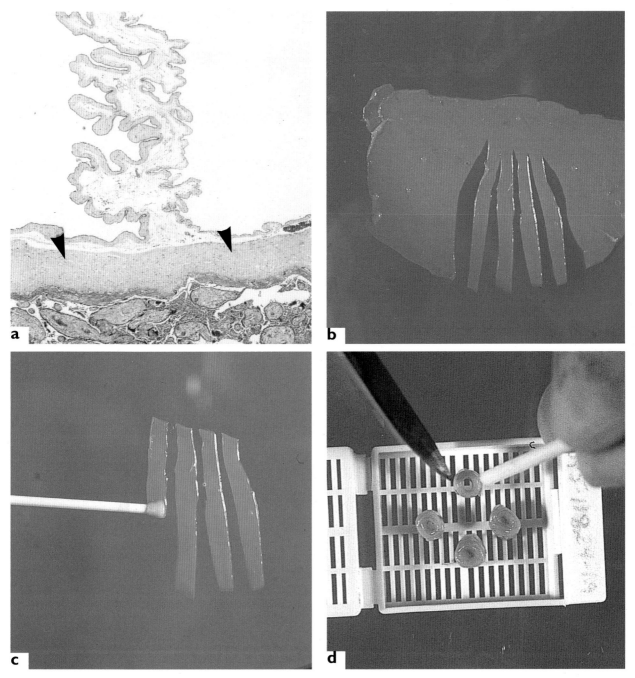

Figure 4.3 Establishing proof of septal status in MC placentas:

(a) Histology (high-power view; H & E stain) of septum from an MC placenta shows the lack of chorion in the septum. The chorionic plate (arrows) runs across the placenta beneath the septum without interruption. The amnion has a complex structure with epithelial and connective tissue components. Such sections are frequently unsatisfactory. A better means of confirming septal status is to prepare membrane rolls (b–d);

(b) To prepare a membrane roll, a portion of the unseparated septum is laid on a firm surface and 4 mm-wide strips are cut;

(c) The strips are separated and rolled up, using the end of a cotton-tipped swab;

(d) The rolls are placed end-on in the cassette;

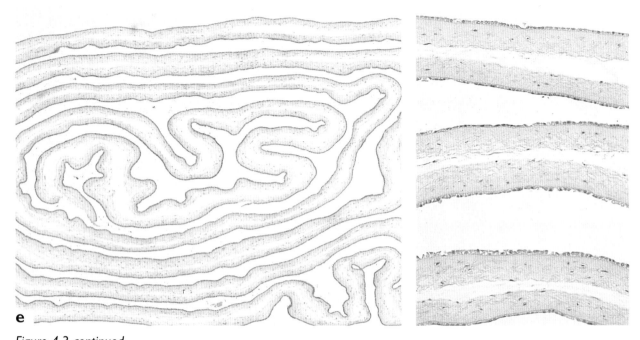

Figure 4.3 continued

(e) Histological views (low power, left; high power, right; H & E) of a septal membrane roll show the multiple components of each amnion and the lack of chorion

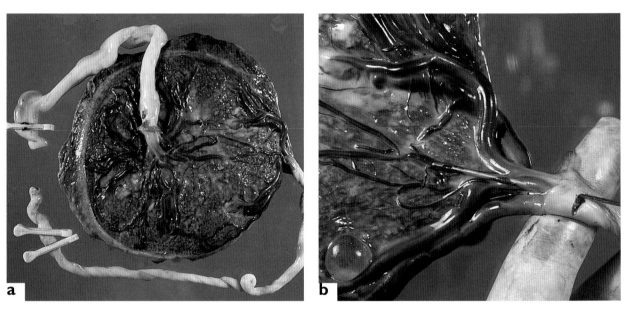

Figure 4.4 Vascular injection studies in MC placentas:

(a) Placenta with evidence of growth discordance: Twin B (with two clamps) has a thin, marginally inserted, cord; twin A weighed 2645 g and twin B weighed 2460 g. If TTT had occurred, twin B would presumably have been the donor.

Injection studies are carried out to document types of vascular anastomoses and extents of unequal venous perfusion:

(b) A cut is made through a selected vessel within 2–3 cm of the cord insertion. With this artery, a probe serves as a dilator;

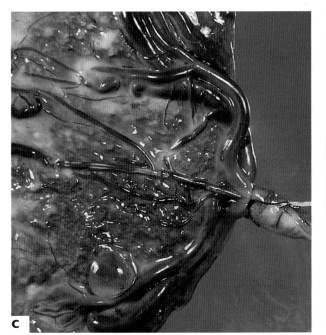

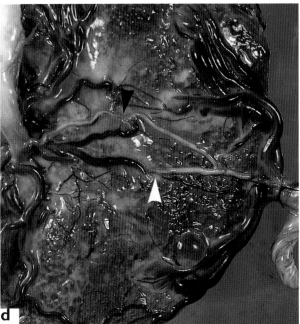

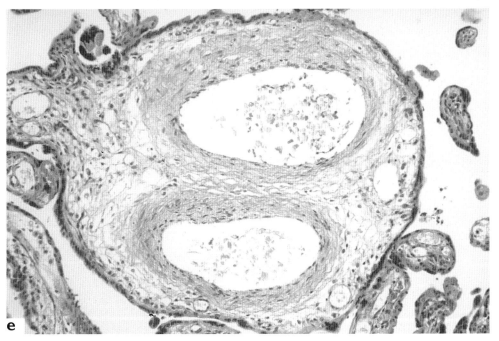

(c) An arterial catheter is inserted and the tip advanced as far as possible towards the potential anastomotic zones. The catheters are tied in place to prevent back-flow;

(d) Yellow dye injected into the artery shows an a↔a anastomosis (black arrow) as well as a zone of potential a→v transfusion (white arrow) from twin B to twin A. The presence of the a↔a anastomosis prevents the development of TTT, but there is clearly unequal venous sharing (A < B), accounting for the a→v zone as well as the growth discordance;

(e) Histology (H & E) shows a cross-section of a stem villus. Yellow dye particles were injected into an umbilical artery of a TTT donor, and blue particles were infused into the vein of the recipient. This villus is clearly in the arteriovenous transfusion zone which caused the TTT, as both dyes from both vascular systems are present

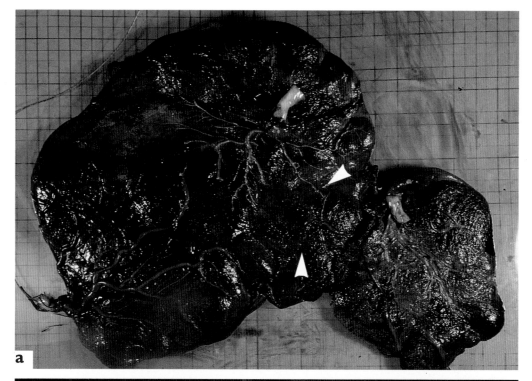

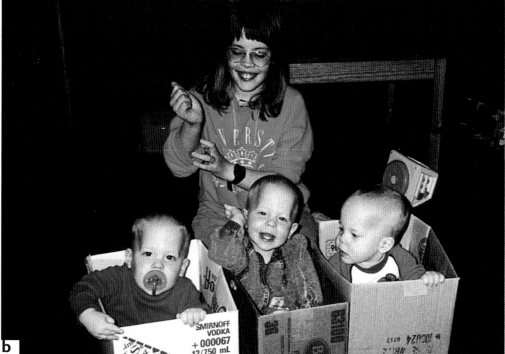

Figure 4.5 Examination of MC triamniotic (TA) triplet placentas:
(a) This MC, TA placenta shows a↔a anastomoses (arrows) among all three triplets. There was no TTT;
(b) The resultant MZ triplets, shown with their older sister;

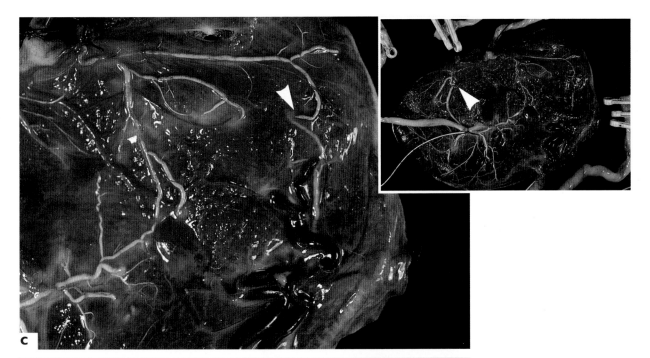

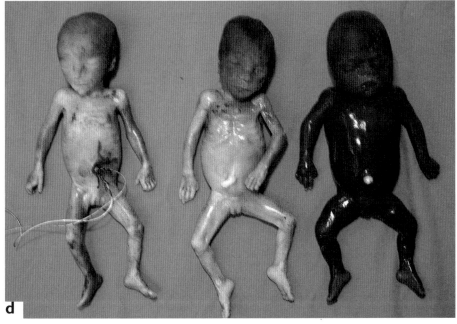

(c) (Inset) This MC, TA placentation resulted in the death of two of the triplets from antenatal TTT. The arteries and vein of triplet B (upper; two clamps) are dyed yellow and purple, respectively. There is an a↔a anastomosis (arrow) with triplet A (lower left; one clamp), and triplet C (lower right; three clamps) has a large and deeply congested cord. (Main picture) A vein (dyed green) of triplet C receives perfused blood from a zone supplied arterially (yellow) by triplet B (arrow). The arteries of triplet C are engorged with blood and triplet A has communications with triplet C. Thus, triplet B is the donor and triplet C is the recipient;

(d) The triplets were delivered at 20 weeks of gestation after onset of acute hydramnios, ruptured membranes and premature labor. Triplet A (left) was 'innocently' involved, triplet B (center) was the donor, and triplet C (right) was the recipient

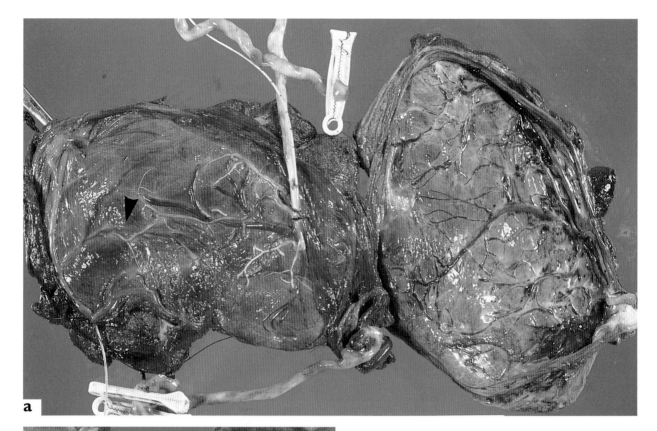

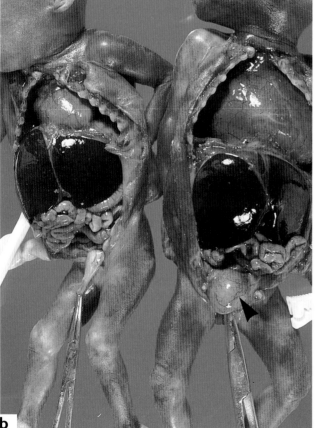

Figure 4.6 Examination of DC triplet placentas: By defintion, these triplet placentas contain an MC twin placenta. The DC placenta may or may not be MZ to the MC twin pair;

(a) These triplets have an MC placenta (left) and a separate (DC) placenta (right). The MC placenta has a zone of a→v anastomosis (arrow) causing antepartum TTT. The artery of the donor (right) MC twin is dyed yellow, and the congested vein of the recipient (left) is green. The DC triplet placenta (on the far right) is separate and is as large as the placenta of the twins;

(b) The MC twins died of antenatal TTT. The congested recipient (who had cardiomegaly, hepatomegaly and a large bladder; arrow) is on the right;

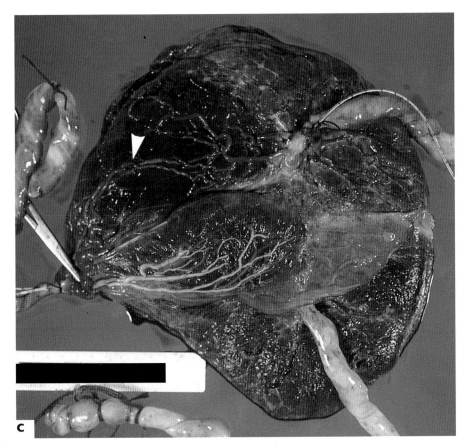

Figure 4.6 continued

(c) In another case, the DC placenta (lower) is fused to the MC placenta, which has a single large a↔a anastomosis (dyed red; arrow)

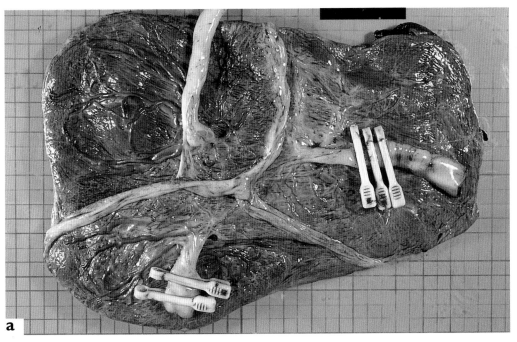

Figure 4.7 Examination of trichorionic (TC) triplet placentas: By definition, TC triplet placentas do not contain MC placentas (but this does not exclude monozygosity);

(a) A fused TC, TA placenta;

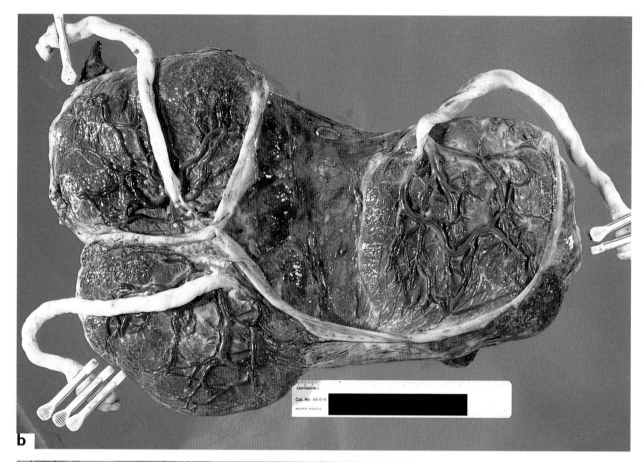

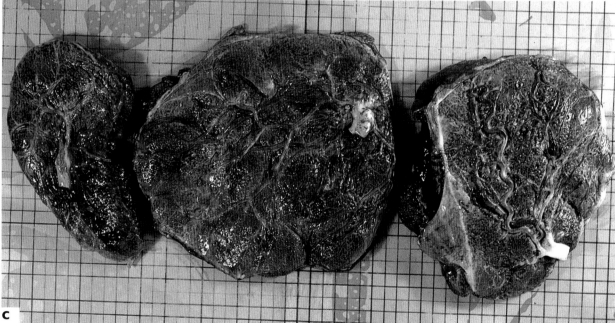

Figure 4.7 continued
(b) In this example, two of the placentas are fused and the third is separate;
(c) Separate TC triplet placentas. The triplets were MZ by DNA VNTR testing

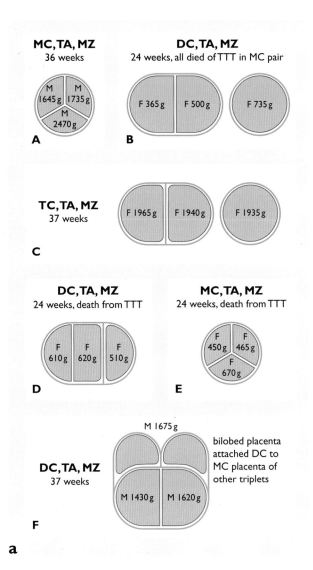

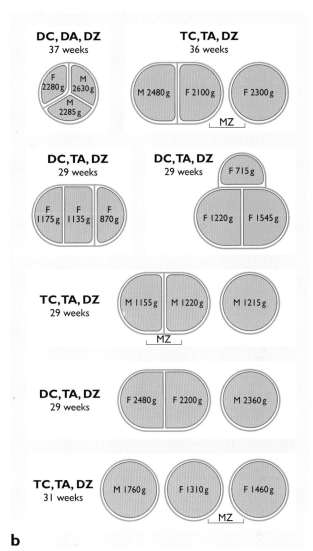

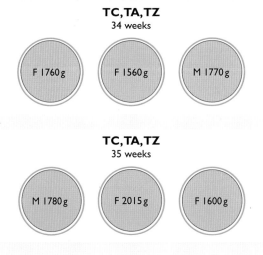

Figure 4.8 Schematic diagrams showing the placentation found in 15 sets of naturally conceived triplets. The triplets were analyzed by placentation, zygosity and outcome:

(a) There were six MZ sets, of which two (sets A and E) were MC, TA. Set A survived (see Figures 4.5 a & b) whereas set E died due to antenatal TTT (see Figures 4.5 c & d). Set D (MC placenta and separate DC placenta for third MZ triplet) is also shown in Figures 4.6 a & b);

(b) Seven sets contained a pair of MZ twins and a DZ co-triplet. Outcomes were generally favorable, and there were only four pairs of MC twins;

(c) The two TZ sets each had separate TC, TA placentation

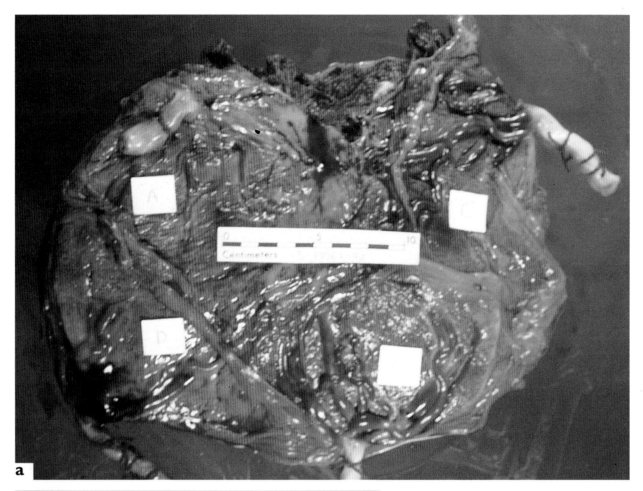

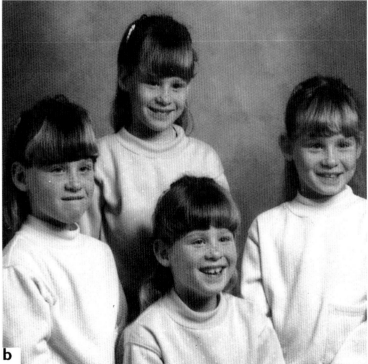

Figure 4.9 Examination of quadruplet placentation:

(a) This placenta was MC and quadra-amniotic (MC, QA). Thus, the quadruplets (see b) were MZ. There was an a↔a anastomosis between quadruplets B and C;

(b) The quadruplets were born at 34 weeks of gestation and were intact

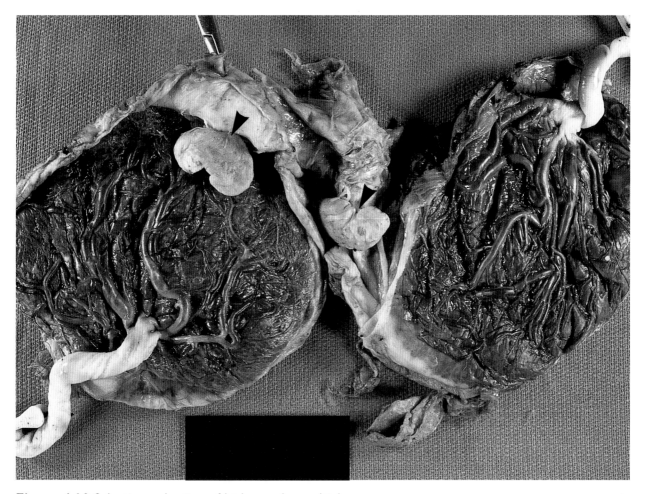

Figure 4.10 Selective reduction of higher-order multiple pregnancy:
The ovulation-induced quintuplet pregnancy was reduced to twins. Two of the three papyraceous fetuses (arrows) can be seen

Part II, Section 2 How to test twins for zygosity

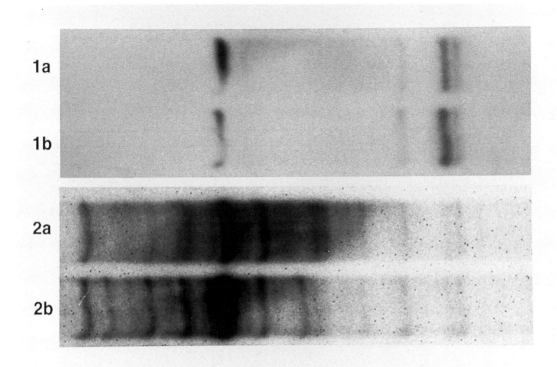

Figure 5.1 Single (high-stringency) and multiple (low-stringency) locus VNTR analysis of twin zygosity: Electrophoretic gel of DNA from DZ twins probed with 3′HVR. For each twin pair, lanes a and b refer to each twin of the pair. By chance, there is apparent monozygosity at high stringency because of the small number of alleles tested (lanes 1a and 1b). Dizygosity is demonstrated using the same probe at low stringency (lanes 2a and 2b)

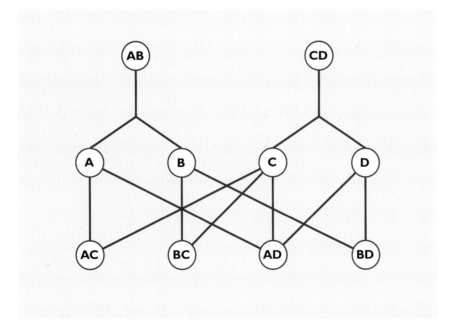

Figure 5.2 Schematic diagram showing the chances that DZ twins will be identical for alleles at a single locus when their parents have four different alleles at that locus: If each parent contributes four alleles for a given gene locus (A, B, C and D), there is a 1:4 possibility that DZ twins will inherit the same pattern of alleles

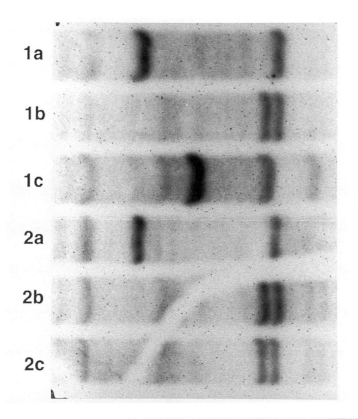

Figure 5.3 Contamination by maternal DNA leads to problems in interpretation: DNA digests from naturally conceived DC, TA triplets, a set in which triplet A (lanes 1a and 2a) was DC to a pair of twins (triplets B and C; lanes 1b and 2b, and lanes 1c and 2c, respectively), who were MC, DA. When chorionic tissues were probed with YNH24 (lanes 1a–1c), there was an apparently TZ pattern. However, analysis of the three amnions with the same probe (lanes 2a–2c) showed that triplet A was DZ to triplets B and C, who were confirmed as MZ. The likely cause of the error with chorion analysis was maternal decidual contamination of the chorion sample of either triplet B or C

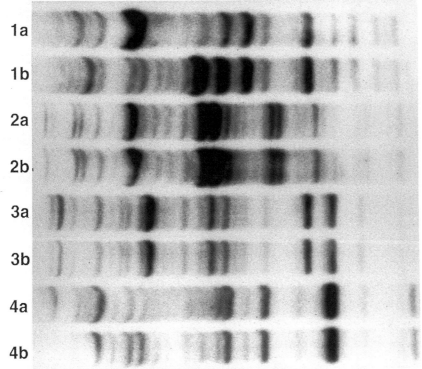

Figure 5.4 Zygosity testing using probes 3'HVR, YNH24 and HMF-1:
(a) Using the 3'HVR probe to analyze DNA from four twin pairs, pairs 1 and 4 proved to be DZ, and pairs 2 and 3 were MZ;

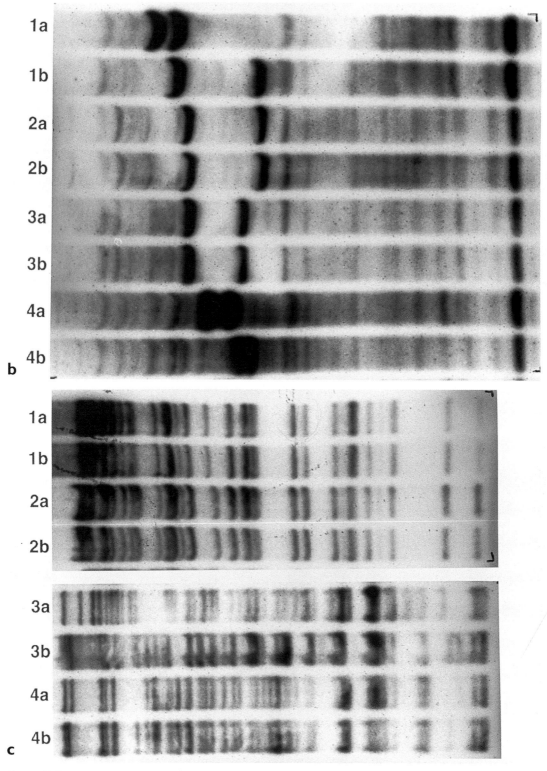

Figure 5.4 continued

(b) Using the YNH24 probe on the same twin pairs confirmed the results;

(c) If the analyses using the 3'HVR and YNH24 probes are inconclusive, then the HMF-I probe can be used. In this gel, twins pairs I and 2 are MZ, and twins pairs 3 and 4 are DZ

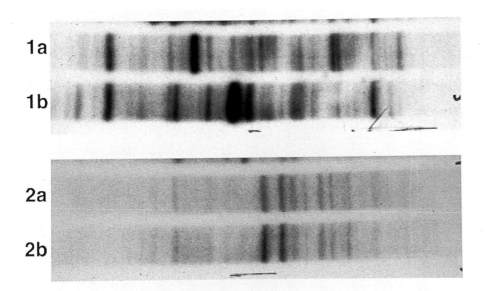

Figure 5.5 A chance pseudo-MZ by one probe analysis leads to problems in interpretation: Lanes 1 a and 1 b show DNA from DZ twins, which was confirmed by the 3′HVR probe. By chance, the YNH24 probe (lanes 2 a and 2 b) gave an apparently MZ result

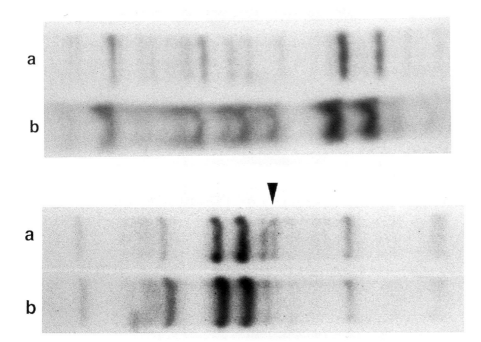

Figure 5.6 Partial DNA digestion leads to problems in interpretation:
   (upper) Using a 3′HVR probe, a partial restriction enzyme digest from one of a pair of twins (lane b) has altered DNA migration during electrophoresis. Repeat analysis showed that the twins were MZ;
   (lower) Anomalous bands (lane a, arrowed) in DNA probed with 3′HVR were caused by partial digestion. Repeat analysis showed that the twins were MZ

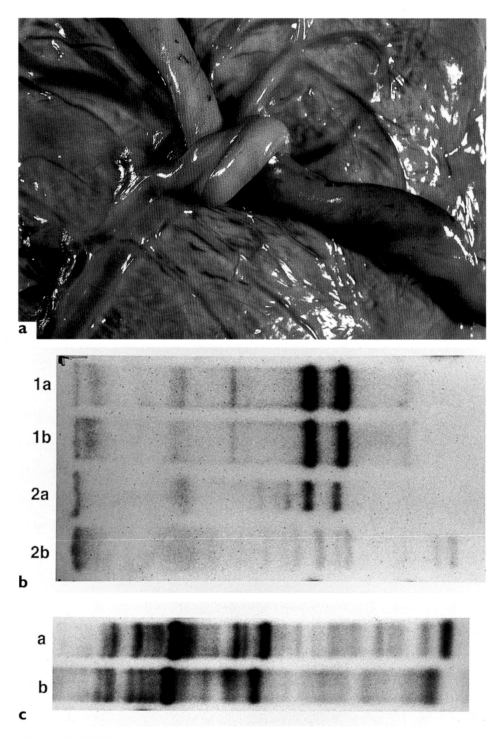

Figure 5.7 DNA degradation leads to problems in interpretation:

(a) Placenta from MC, MA twins shows cord entanglement causing fetal death of twin B;

(b) DNA extracted from chorion (lanes 1a and 1b) is well preserved and confirms monozygosity using the YNH24 probe. DNA from the necrotic cord of twin B (lane 2b) shows anomalous migration and extra bands compared with DNA from the surviving twin (lane 2a);

(c) Electrophoretic migration of DNA from a pair of twins probed with YNH24 shows DNA degradation in lane b. Subsequent analysis showed that the twins were MZ

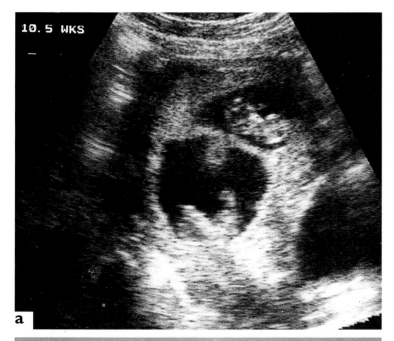

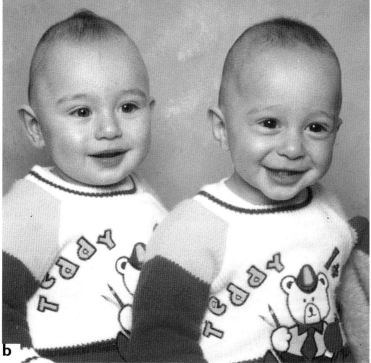

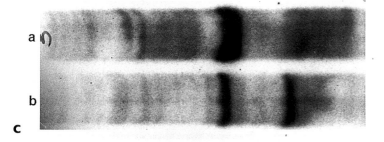

Figure 5.8 Zygosity analysis of phenotypically similar DZ twins:

(a) Ultrasonogram of DC twins taken at 10 weeks;

(b) At birth and for several years, the boys were strikingly similar in phenotype;

(c) DNA probed with YNH24 at low stringency showed that the twins are clearly DZ

Part II, Section 3 How to photograph twin faces for medical purposes

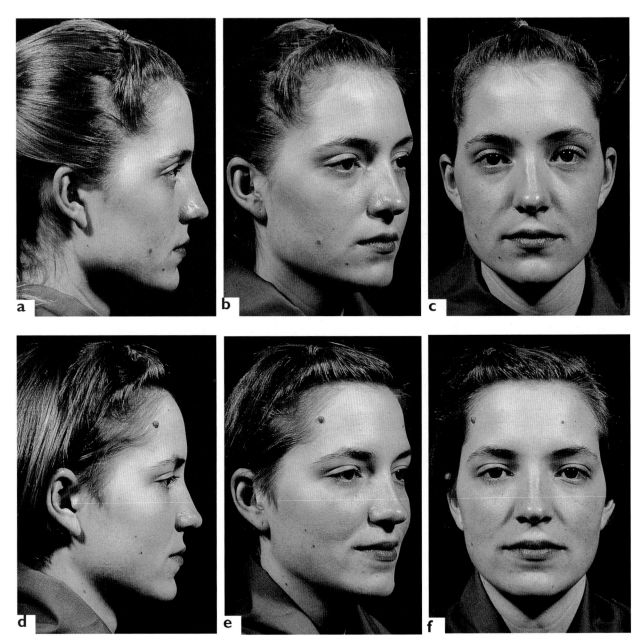

Figure 6.1 Standard images of a pair of female MZ twins: Right profile; right anterior oblique; frontal (a–c, twin A; d–f, twin B). Note the uneven development of nevi in the two women (*continued on facing page*)

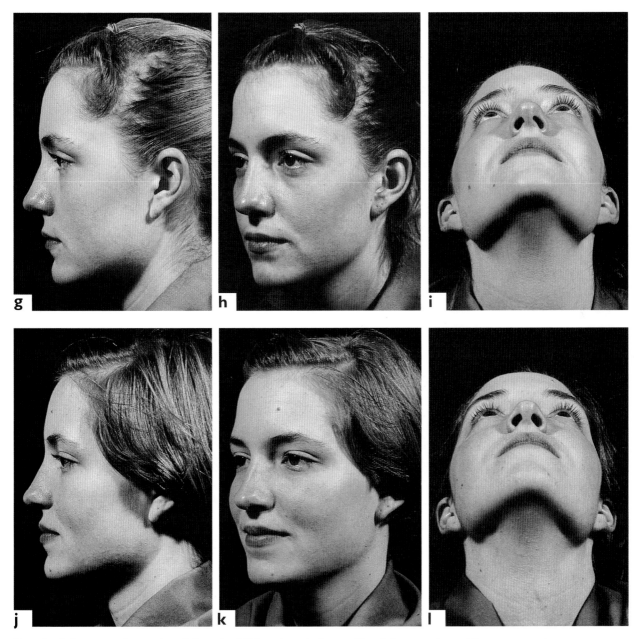

Standard images of a pair of female MZ twins: Left profile; left anterior oblique; worm's-eye view (g–i, twin A; j–l, twin B). Note the uneven development of nevi in the two women. In addition, twin A has a peaked left nostril whereas twin B has symmetrical nostrils

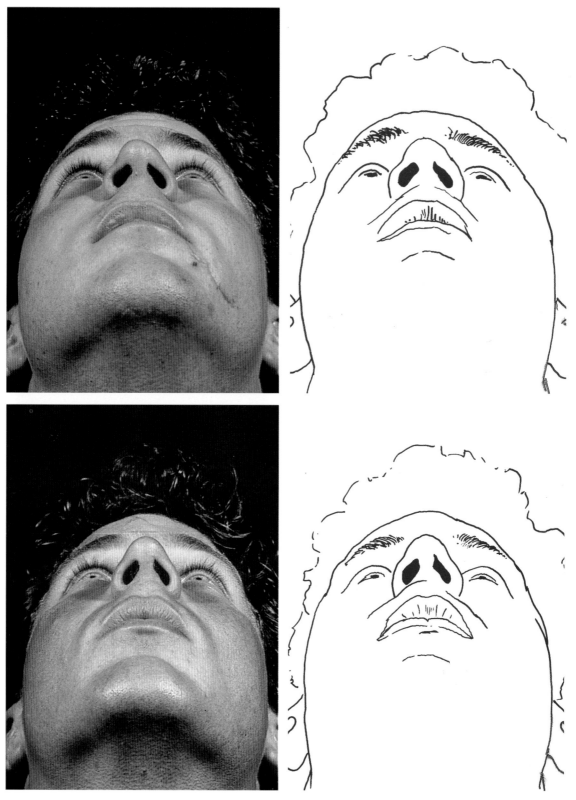

Figure 6.2 Twins A (upper) and B (lower) shown in worm's-eye view. The left nostrils of both twins are peaked and asymmetrical, as emphasized in the accompanying line drawings

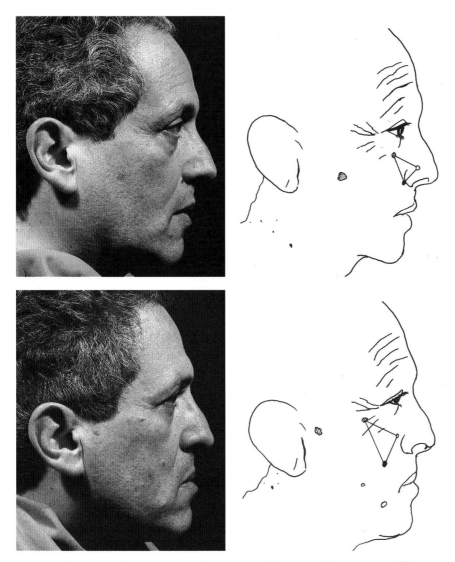

Figure 6.3 Detailed analysis of skin wrinkling and lesions in MZ twins (right profiles). Both twins have six primary forehead creases, three curving upwards, and three sloping downwards as 'crow's-feet' near the lateral canthus. Both twins also have a single crease of the earlobe, and a single wrinkle projecting downwards where the helix of the ear joins the temple. Their skin lesions also show near concordance. Twin A (upper) has a well-defined seborrheic keratosis 3.5 cm anterior to the ear. Twin B (lower) has a similar lesion, but only 1.5 cm anterior to the ear, suggesting that the precursor cells for this benign neoplasm have not migrated as far anteriorly during embryological development. Both twins have three intradermal nevi on the upper cheek: the uppermost have patchy pigmentation; the anterior-most are hypopigmented; and the lowermost are hyperpigmented. However, twin B also has two hypopigmented nevi on the cheek which are not apparent on twin A. All lesions appear to lie more anteriorly in twin A than in twin B. Another difference is seen in the cluster of lentigos on the neck just below the ear: twin A has one large and four small lesions whereas twin B has one large and three small lesions

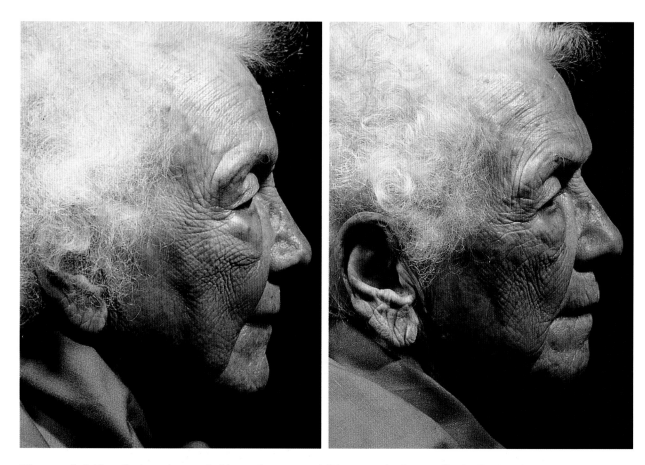

Figure 6.4 Detailed analysis of the eyebrows in MZ twins (right profiles). Each of these sisters has just begun to develop gray hairs in their eyebrows, as evidenced by the same two gray hairs in the same eyebrow. The analysis shows that the depigmentation of hair as an aging phenomenon is precisely timed and affects specific hair follicles in a clear pattern. Regarding the extent to which genetics is involved in aging, there appears to be control of timing and topography to an unexpected degree

Part III Lives of some twins and their parents

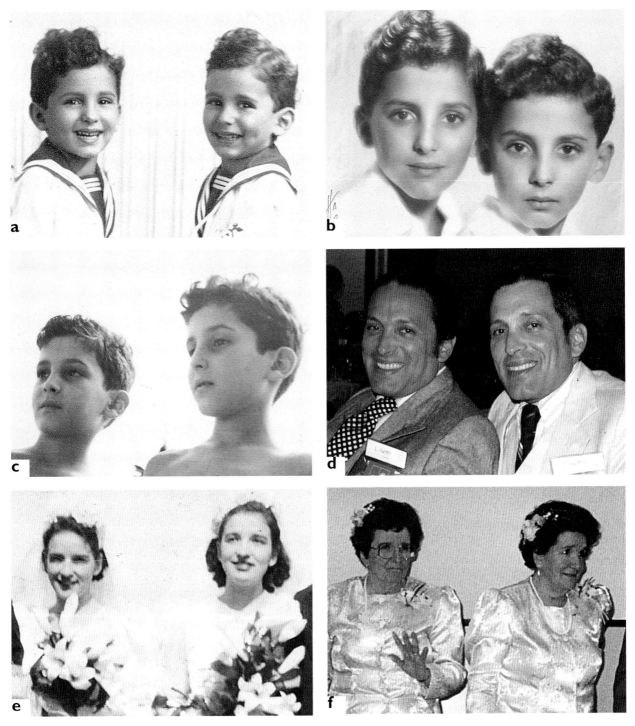

Figure 7.1 Life-long phenotypic resemblances in three MZ twin pairs:
(a–d) Louis Keith and his brother Donald erroneously believed, for many years, that they were DZ because they were DC and not absolutely 'identical';
(e & f) MZ twin sisters at their wedding and their golden-wedding celebrations;

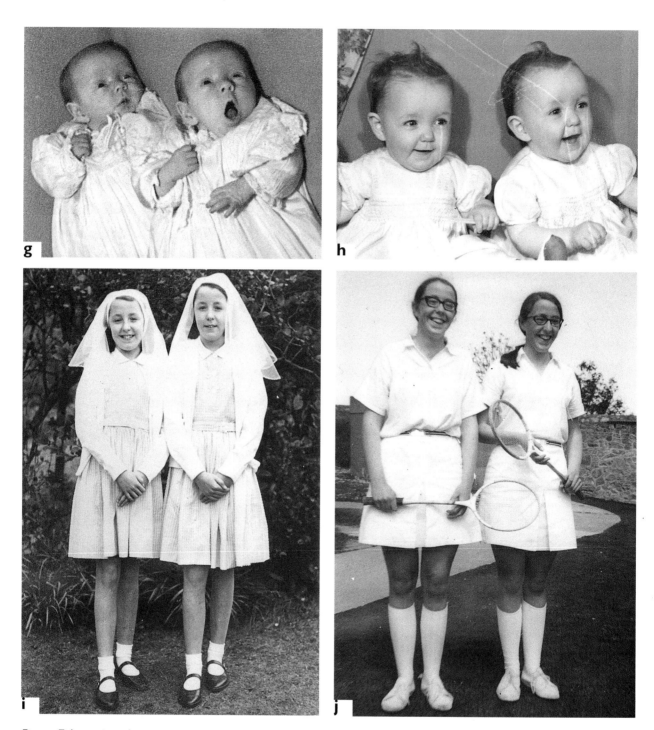

Figure 7.1 continued

(g–l) MZ twin sisters who were uncertain of their zygosity until they underwent DNA VNTR testing. They are shown here at ages 5 weeks, 1 year, 11 years, 16 years, 28 years and 41 years. Note their opposite-handedness (j);

In all three pairs of twins, the phenotypic resemblances have remained strong throughout life. The twins and their parents themselves can usually see differences whereas others may not be able to distinguish between the twins. This causes difficulty in understanding the difference between being 'identical' and being MZ

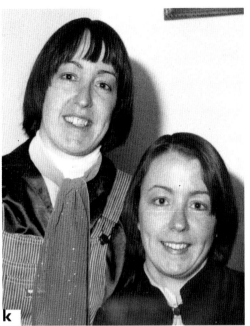

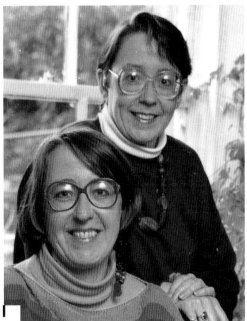

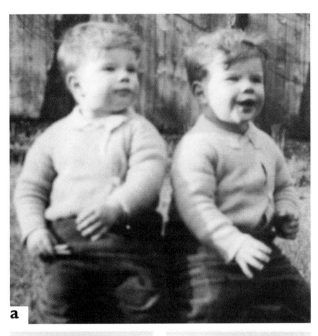

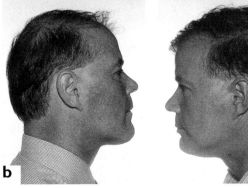

Figure 7.2 Medical implications of monozygosity: These twins decided that they were DZ because of phenotypic differences (see page 72). Note the suggestion of mirroring in their postures. One twin received a renal transplant from the other and was treated with immunosuppression for 15 years before it was recognized that the twins were, in fact, MZ.

(a) The twins are opposite-handed, leading to a mirror-like body language;

(b) The twins have opposite occipital hair-whorls. In most other respects, however, they are strikingly similar, although the twin on the left shows the effects of long-term steroids and cytotoxic drugs

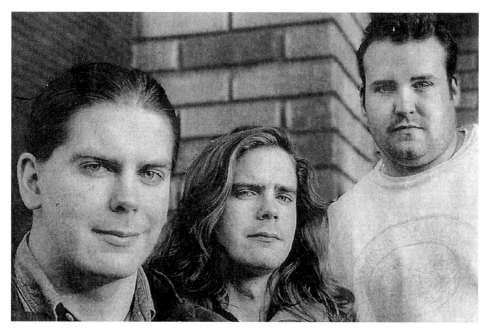

Figure 7.3 Personal implications of chorionicity and zygosity: These three boys (an MZ twin pair and a singleton) were mistakenly identified and named when they were in the newborn nursery (see page 73). The boy in the middle and the one on the right were raised as a DZ twin pair (because their placentas were DC), but it was subsequently discovered that the boy in the middle and the one on the left were, in fact, the MZ, DC twins. Despite the different hairstyles, their facial appearances are clearly similar

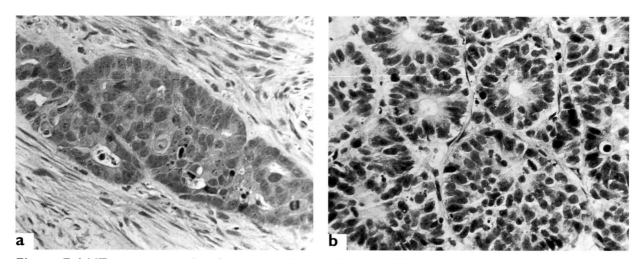

Figure 7.4 MZ twins concordant for genetic disease: A pair of MZ twins both had a form of congenital antibody deficiency, specifically, hyper-IgM hypogammaglobulinemia (autosomal-recessive). This is often complicated by the development of liver cancer in the second decade of life. Twin A presented with widespread intra-abdominal malignancy and died shortly thereafter at age 24 years. His MZ twin (B) was extensively investigated at the time of twin A's illness, but no disease was found. However, there was a rapid onset of similar disease 1 year later.
(a) Liver needle biopsy from twin A shows widespread infiltrating cancer;
(b) Similar appearances in a liver biopsy of twin B taken 1 year later

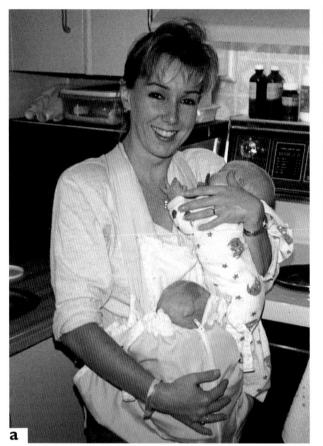

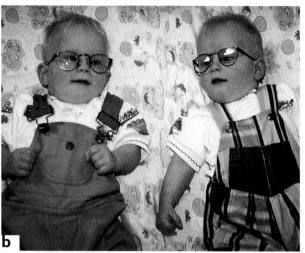

Figure 7.5 Survivors of TTT, but with residual problems:

(a) Claudine and her twins at age 13 weeks (see pages 73–75). The twins needed to be carried constantly to prevent their frequent bouts of crying;

(b) Michel and Mathieu at age 1 year

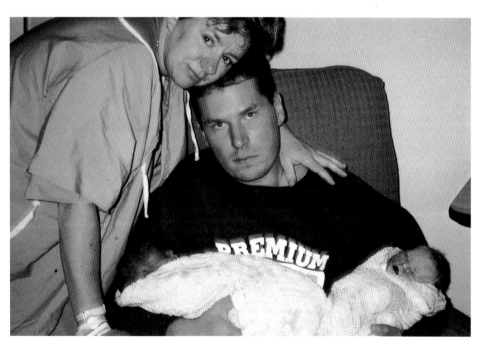

Figure 7.6 Stillborn fetuses due to acute perinatal TTT: Susan comforts Dale, who carries Nicole (on the left; as the recipient, she was deeply congested) and Katie (see pages 75–77)

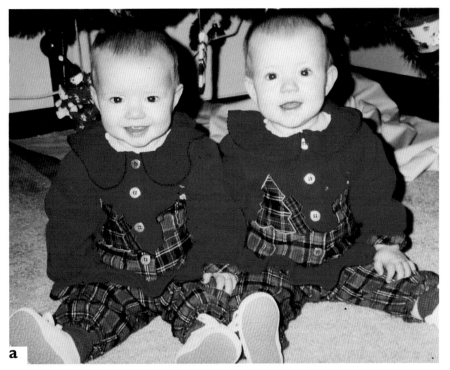

Figure 7.7 Fetoscopic laser coagulation treatment of chronic antenatal TTT:

(a) Amanda (left) and Christine (right) at age 7 months were successfully treated after early antenatal diagnosis of TTT;

(b) Their placenta shows multiple areas of coagulation along the equator. There is unequal venous sharing favoring Christine, the recipient. Coagulation (arrows) separated the two circulations;

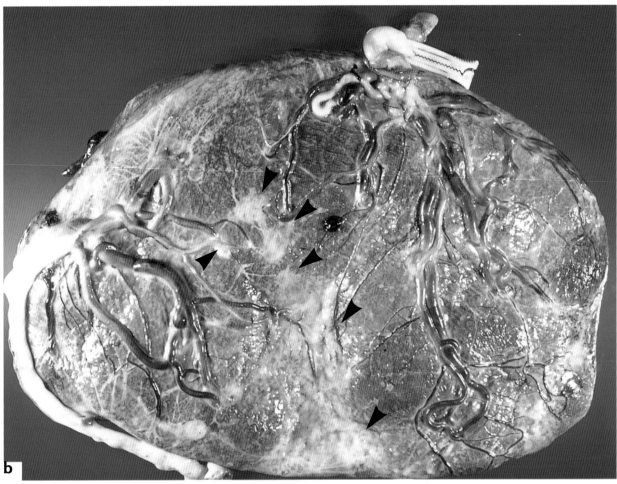

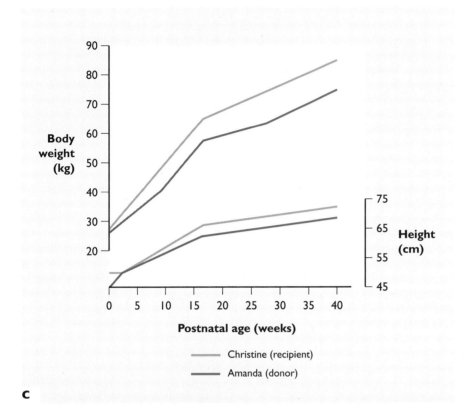

(c) Graph showing the postnatal growth of the twins

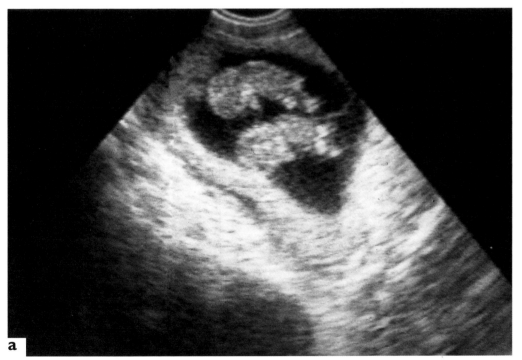

Figure 7.8 Ultrasonograms showing early antenatal diagnosis of TTT (same case as in Figure 7.7):

(a) Ultrasonogram at 10 weeks shows twins with a thin septal membrane, indicating MC, DA placentation, but no apparent growth discordance.

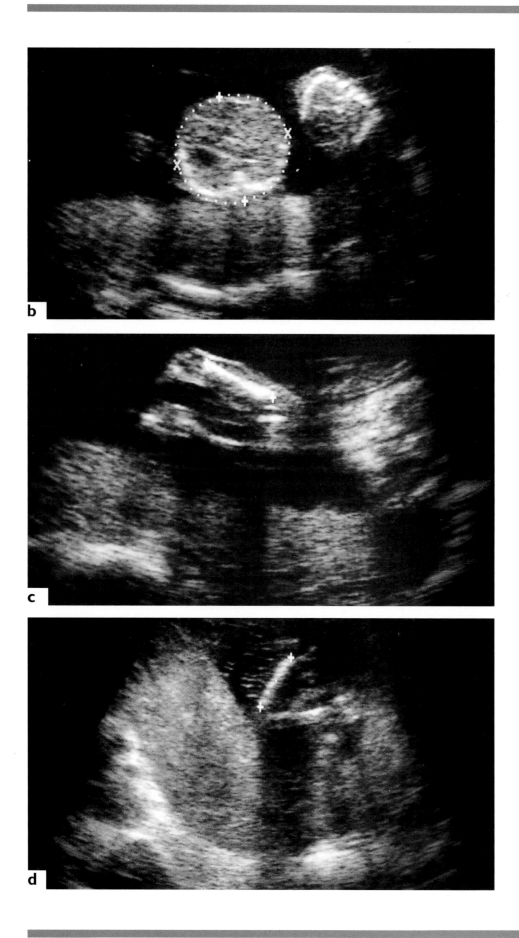

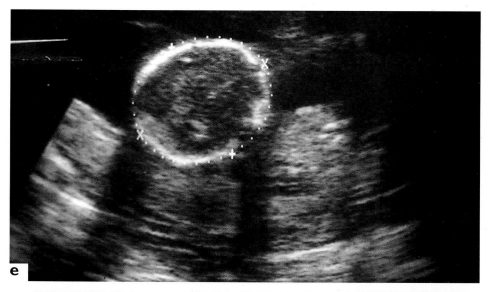

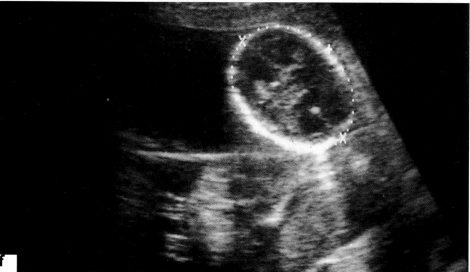

Figure 7.8 continued

(b) Ultrasonograms were taken at 18 weeks because the fundal height was that usually seen at 27 weeks. Significant growth discordance with polyhydramnios / oligohydramnios can now be seen. The abdominal circumference of the recipient was 122 mm;

(c) The recipient's femoral length was 26 mm;

(d) The donor's femoral length was 20 mm;

(e) The recipient's head circumference was 146 mm, with a biparietal diameter of 39 mm;

(f) The donor's head circumference was 133 mm, with a biparietal diameter of 34 mm and dolichocephaly secondary to oligohydramnios. There was now a 10-day discordance in the calculated gestational ages of the twins

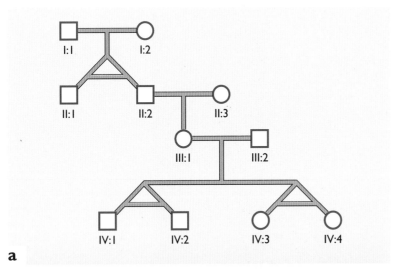

a

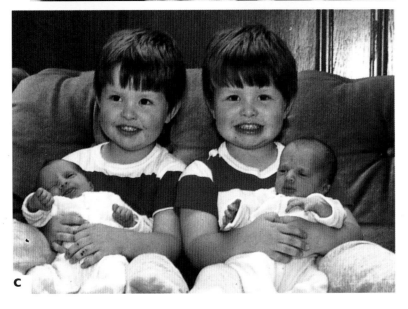

b

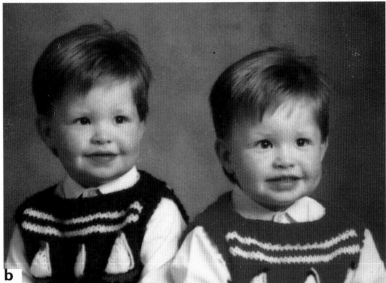

c

Figure 7.9 Familial MZ twinning: Family 1 (a–f); Family 2 (g–k) and Family 3 (l–q).

(a) Pedigree of Family 1;

(b) A mother (III:1) had a pair of MZ boys (IV:1&2) in her first pregnancy;

(c) Her second pregnancy resulted in MZ twin girls (IV:3&4);

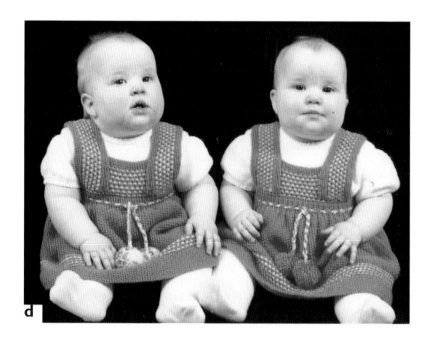

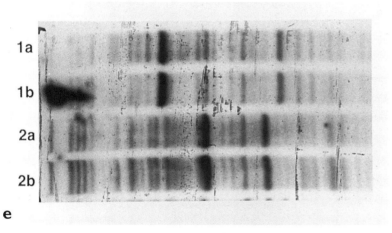

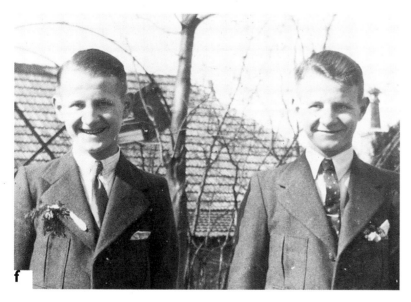

(d) These girls are shown here at age 1 year;

(e) DNA from the boys (lanes 1a and 1b) and the girls (lanes 2a and 2b) were probed with 3'HVR, and both sets proved to be MZ;

(f) The mother's father (II:2) is one of MZ twins (II:1 & 2) and was also confirmed by DNA testing.;

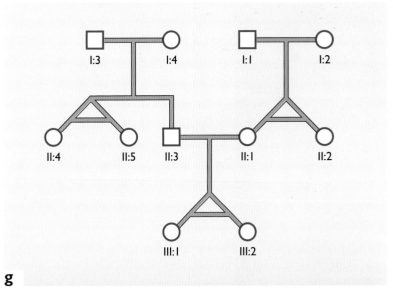

g

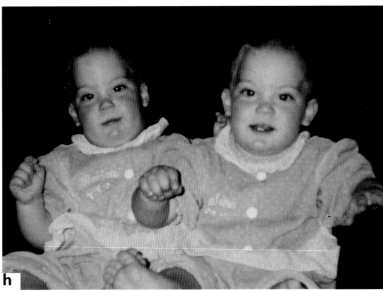

h

Figure 7.9 continued
    (g) Pedigree of Family 2;
    (h) In this family, there was a pair of MZ twin girls (III : 1 & 2);

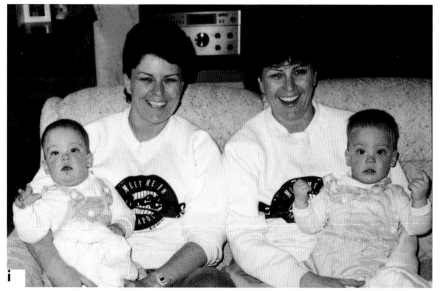

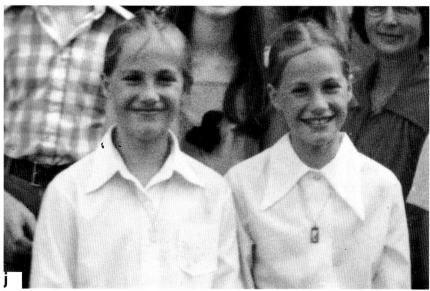

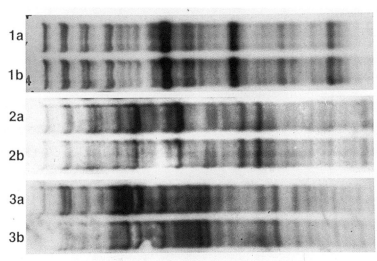

(i) The girls are shown here with their mother and aunt, who are also MZ twins (II : 1 & 2);

(j) The girls' father (II : 3) has MZ twin sisters (II : 4 & 5);

(k) DNA samples were probed with 3'HVR: Lanes 1a and 1b are from the girls (III : 1 & 2); lanes 2a and 2b are from the girls' mother and her MZ twin sister (II : 1 & 2); lanes 3a and 3b are from the girls' paternal MZ twin aunts (II : 4 & 5);

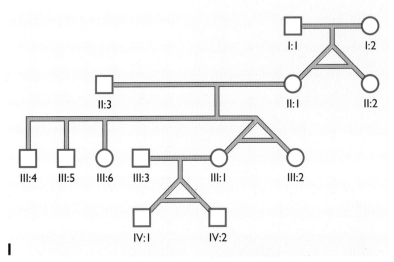

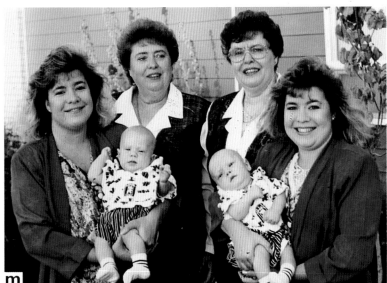

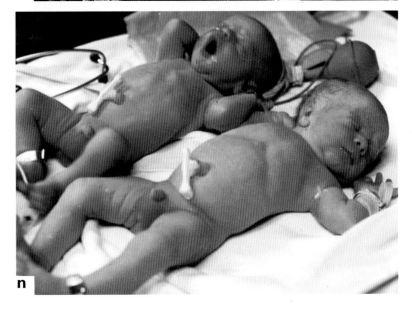

Figure 7.9 continued

(l) Pedigree of Family 3 shows MZ twinning in three successive generations;

(m) The boys (IV:1 & 2) were MC, as were their mother (III:1) and her MZ twin sister (III:2). The mother of the twin sisters (II:1) is one of MZ twins (II:1 & 2), but their chorionicity is unknown;

(n) The boys (IV:1 & 2) had acute TTT at birth without growth discordance;

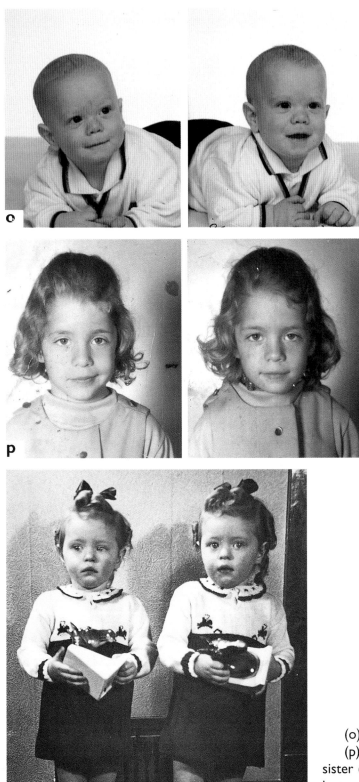

(o) The boys at age 9 months;

(p) The mother of the boys with her MZ twin sister (III : 1 & 2) at age 5 years. One of them (III : 2) has severe scoliosis and congenital heart disease;

(q) The oldest pair of MZ twins (II : 1 & 2) at 2 years of age

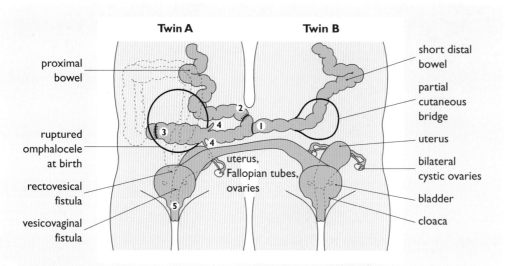

a

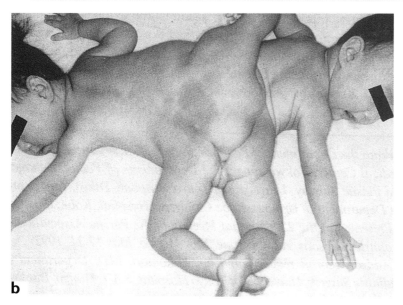

b

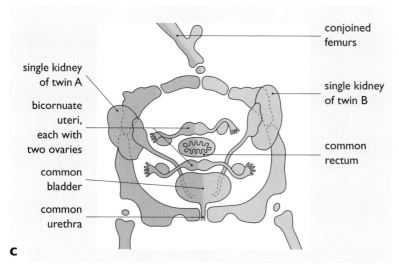

c

Figure 7.10 Postpartum surgical management of conjoined twins:

(a) Case 1: Diagram of the anatomy of omphalopagus twins (see page 79);

(b) Case 2: Asymmetrical female ischiopagus twins (see page 79);

(c) Diagram detailing the separation of the ischiopagus twins shown in **b**;

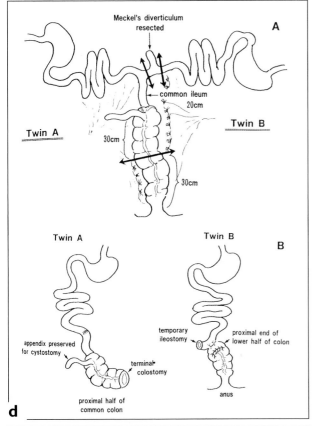

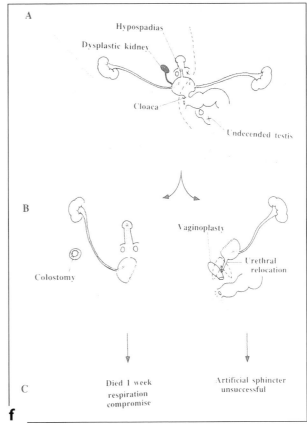

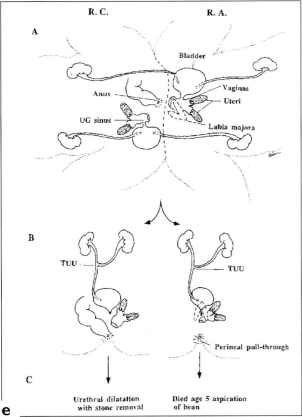

(d) Another diagram detailing the separation of the ischiopagus twins shown in **b**;

(e) Case 3: Diagram detailing separation of symmetrical female ischiopagus twins (see page 80);

(f) Case 4: Diagram detailing separation of asymmetrical male ischiopagus twins (see page 80);

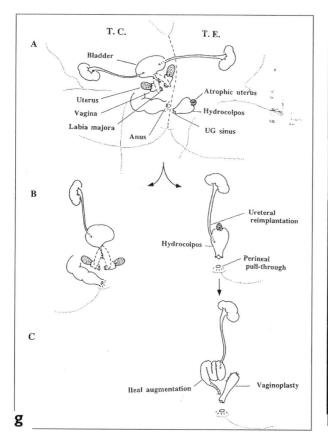

g

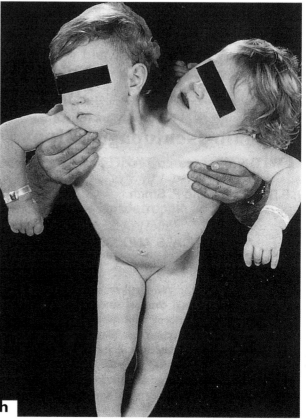

h

i

Figure 7.10 continued

(g) Case 5: Diagram detailing separation of asymmetrical male ischiopagus twins (see page 80);

(h) Case 6: Female dicephalic twins (see page 80);

(i) Diagram detailing separation of the twins shown in (h);

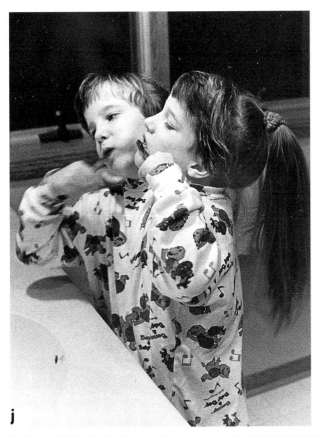

(j) Female dicephalic conjoined twins who have not been surgically separated (see page 80)

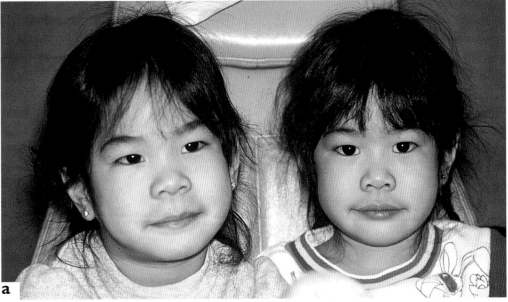

Figure 7.11 Mirroring and apparent mirroring in MZ twins: Many parents of twins believe their twins show mirroring phenomena. The case here shows how complex and interesting mirroring may be from a developmental point of view:

(a) These twin girls were proved to be MZ by VNTR zygosity testing. The mother noticed that they appeared to have mirror-image dental abnormalities, with fusion of one pair of lower lateral incisor and canine teeth, but on opposite sides of the mouth;

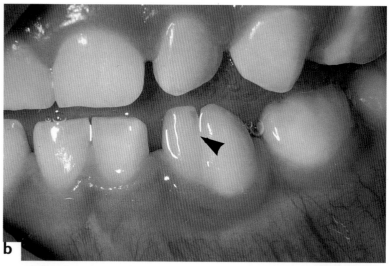

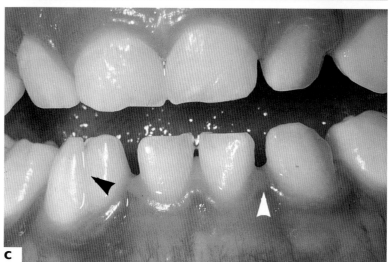

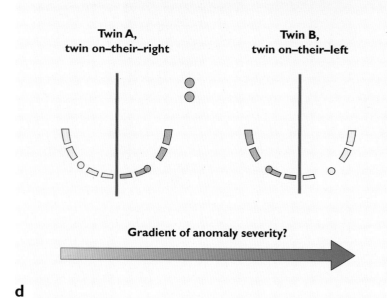

Twin A,
twin on–their–right

Twin B,
twin on–their–left

Gradient of anomaly severity?

d

Figure 7.11 continued

(b) Twin A (upper) has fusion on the left (arrow);

(c) Twin B (lower) has fusion on the right (black arrow). However, this twin also has complete absence of the left lower lateral incisor (white arrow); thus, this is not an example of true mirroring;

(d) Schematic diagram showing how, instead of mirroring, the twins may be showing 'increasing severity' of a dental abnormality, moving from the right side of one twin to the left side of the other. This suggests an entirely different developmental mechanism for this anomaly

Acknowledgements

The authors are grateful to the following authors, journals, colleagues, twins and parents of twins for their kind permission to reproduce many of the illustrations included in this book. (Some of the figures have never been published before and are marked with an asterisk.)

Dr John Marlow (page 95, upper right)

Part I, Section 1
Americal Journal of Medical Genetics (Figures 1.8 & 1.9)

Part I, Section 2
Keith LG, Papiernik E, Keith DM, *et al.*, eds. *Multiple Pregnancy: Epidemiology, Gestation & Perinatal Outcome.* Carnforth: Parthenon Publishing, 1995:196 (Figures 2.1 b & 2.2 b)

Dr AB Kurtz and *Radiology* (Figures 2.1 c–e & 2.2 c)

Dr Regina Robinson (Figure 2.3 a)*

Dr Richard P Perkins and *Obstetrics and Gynecology* (Figure 2.3 b)

Dr J Leveaucoupet and *Pediatric Radiology* (Figure 2.5)

Rosa de Vermette, Professor Carl Nimrod and Dr Karen Ash (Figures 2.6–2.8 & 2.9 e)*

Dr GA Aisenbrey and *Obstetrics and Gynecology* (Figure 2.9 a)

Dr MA Belfort and *American Journal of Obstet-rics and Gynecology* (Figures 2.9 b–d)

Dr T Westover and *Obstetrics and Gynecology* (Figures 2.10 & 2.11)

Dr Nestor Demianczuk (Figure 2.12)*

Dr Laurence Devoe and *Journal of Reproductive Medicine* (Figure 2.13)

Dr GCML Christiaens and *Prenatal Diagnosis* (Figure 2.14)

Dr Keith Still (Figure 2.15)*

Part I, Section 3
American Journal of Medical Genetics (Figure 3.1)

Anonymous and Dr Julian De Lia (Figure 3.9 c & d)*

Anonymous (Figure 3.17 c)*

Mr MR Cox, FRCOG (Figure 3.20 a)*

Anonymous (Figure 3.20 c)*

March of Dimes Birth Defects Foundation (Figure 3.21 a–d, f–h)

Dr Ronan O'Rahilly (Figure 3.21 j & k)*

Dr Nestor Demianczuk (Figure 3.22 a)*

Dr George Vujanic (Figure 3.22 b)*

Dr Samir Amr (Figure 3.22 c)*

Dr Joe Rutledge (Figure 3.22 d)*

National Museum of Anthropology, Mexico City, Mexico (Figure 3.22 e)*

Part II, Section 1
Anonymous (Figure 4.5 b)*

American Journal of Medical Genetics (Figure 4.8)

Anonymous (Figure 4.9 b)*

Part II, Section 2
Anonymous (Figure 5.8 b)*

Part II, Section 3

David Teplica, MD, MFA and The Collected Image, Evanston, IL (Figures 6.1–6.4)

Part III

Louis G and Donald M Keith (Figure 7.1 a–d)*

Anonymous (Figure 7.1 e & f)*

Anonymous (Figure 7.1 g–l)*

Anonymous (Figure 7.2)*

Anonymous (Figure 7.3)*

Anonymous (Figure 7.5)*

Anonymous (Figure 7.6)*

Parents of the twins, Dr Julian De Lia and Dr JH O'Flynn (Figures 7.7 & 7.8)*

Anonymous (Figure 7.9 b–f)*

Anonymous (Figure 7.9 g–k)*

Anonymous (Figure 7.9 l–q)*

Dr Herve Blanchard and *Journal of Pediatric Surgery* (Figure 7.10 a)

Dr Kinji Yokomori and *Journal of Pediatric Surgery* (Figure 7.10 b–d)

Dr John M Duckett and *Journal of Urology* (Figure 7.10 e–g)

Dr Mark Stringer and *Journal of Pediatric Surgery* (Figure 7.10 h & i)

Parents of the twins and Steve Wewerka / Impact Visuals (Figure 7.10 j)

Parents of the twins and *American Journal of Medical Genetics* (Figure 7.11 a–c)

Index